GOING BACK TO ZEN

WHERE TO FIND PEACE
SO YOU CAN LIVE LIKE MAD
Tiny tips for life's different seasons

Copyright 2017 & Design Concept contact@JanineVance.com

2020 UPDATE: These books were written a few years before the covid-culture upheaval and have been updated slightly to allude to the pandemic, but do not address quarantine and isolation procedures as required by any governmental, state, or health agency.

The ideas, procedures, and suggestions contained in *Going Back to Zen* are not intended as a substitute for consulting with your medical healthcare provider. Readers are able to discern for themselves when to seek professional medical care. Neither the author nor publisher shall be liable or responsible for any loss or damage allegedly arising from any information or ideas from this book.

GOING BACK TO ZEN

CONTENTS

INTRODUCTION 4

THE VITAL IMPORTANCE OF YOU 7

IN THE BEGINNING WAS THE "WORD" 11

WORDS ARE ENERGY 17

WHEN THEY ACCUSE YOU OF BEING "BAD" 23

LOVE IS G.O.D 29

UNPLUGGING & BREAKING FREE 33

THE PAIN MIGHT NOT BE IN YOUR HEAD 36

ESSENTIALS FROM MOTHER NATURE 42

TACTICAL BREATHING 50

FOOD IS MEDICINE 56

NEEDLES AND KNOTS 63

HANDS-ON HEALING 68

where to find peace so you can live like mad

HOLDERS OF LIFE KNOWLEDGE 72

MASSAGE FOR THE SOUL 79

A GENTLE, YET POWERFUL HEALER 85

LOST AND FOUND IN THOUGHT 91

CENTERED FOR LIFE 99

MOVE TO IMPROVE 104

TAP INTO YOUR INTUITION 111

STOP AND SMELL THE FLOWERS 114

MORE FROM MOTHER NATURE'S BOUNTY 121

CONCLUSION: GOING FROM RICHES TO RAGS 125

GIFT MEDITATION 133

DEAR GENTLE AND WISE SOUL 136

EXCERPT FROM THE POWER OF ISOLATION 139

ABOUT JANINE VANCE 145

INTRODUCTION

Welcome to *Going Back to Zen: Where to Find Peace So You Can Live Like Mad*. I'm Janine Vance, and I am delighted to share this journey with you. This book is a guide to navigating life's inevitable ups and downs, offering a path to finding joy and tranquility regardless of your circumstances.

Life is full of unexpected twists and turns, and sometimes, we find ourselves transitioning from a state of abundance to one of scarcity. This shift can be disorienting and challenging, but it also presents an opportunity to discover the profound value and joy in the simple, free offerings of the universe and nature.

Especially in today's digital age, social media can feel like an inescapable part of life. It connects us, entertains us, and informs us. However, for many, it can also be a source of stress, anxiety, and even bullying. I know this all too well. I was never a fan of social media and found myself dreading each notification and avoiding my accounts altogether. This experience was a key motivator for writing this book, and I want to share with you how you might find peace if you decide to go back to zen and begin again. Maybe you didn't get attacked on social media; maybe you've lost a job or spent months or even decades trying to accomplish something without success. Perhaps you've been on top of your game for a while or went from being popular to very, very unpopular. This book is intended to help you gain peace while recovering.

GOING BACK TO ZEN

Throughout this book, we explore various themes and interactive elements designed to help you reconnect with yourself, nature, and the world around you. You can embrace these practices and make them a part of your daily life or just use one or two suggestions. You'll find practical tips, meditative practices, and holistic insights designed to help you embrace the beauty of what is freely available to us all. Whether you're basking in the warmth of the sun, feeling the cool breeze on your face, or simply enjoying a quiet moment of reflection, nature provides us with endless treasures that cost nothing but offer everything.

The essence of this book lies in finding peace—a state of mind where "PEACE" stands for People Enjoying A Cohesive Environment. When we cultivate inner peace, we can live with a zest and enthusiasm that transcends material wealth. This peace empowers us to live like mad, passionately and fully, embracing each moment with gratitude and joy.

I've included various themes, from the healing power of words and the importance of self-compassion, to the wonders of natural remedies and the significance of breathing and mindfulness. Each chapter includes interactive elements to help you apply these concepts to your daily life, fostering a deeper connection to yourself and the world around you. As you read and engage with the exercises, I hope you discover the richness of a life rooted in simplicity and mindfulness. May you find strength in the free resources that surround us and joy in the present moment. Remember, true wealth is not measured by material possessions but by the peace and happiness we cultivate within ourselves.

Thank you for joining me on this journey back to zen. Let's embrace the free gifts of the universe, find peace, and live like mad together.

With care and concern,

Janine Vance

THE VITAL IMPORTANCE OF YOU

If you have ever been removed from or deprived of your family, circle of friends, coworkers, or even a beloved community, you probably know how uncertain it can feel to be a bit lonely. Our saving grace becomes our return to oneness. Sometimes leaving our childhood teachings — even if it's only temporary — is the best thing we can do for ourselves. We can use loss as an opportunity to remember from where we originate and become ourselves fully. From this place of fullness, we can reach out to others from a place of holistic health and well-being. All of us humans are birthed from the universe —something so grand, we can't even imagine its power. We are born to two individuals who belong to an extensive line of maternal and paternal lineage, aunts, uncles, and cousins, who spring forth nieces, and nephews. When feeling heavy energy, it helps me to remember that I belong to a universal family line, and not only that, my ancestry is stretched throughout time and everlasting. In fact, it's universal. We come from the stars. Together we exist. Apart from that, we are a great invisible family.

This long ancestry makes us part of an amazing global clan. We might feel alone at times, but from behind the scenes, we are surrounded by essences much larger than we can imagine. This lineage is in our blood, and it is in our chi (our breath of life). It lives in us. We live in it. We are the extension of it: a significant member of this everlasting thread

where to find peace so you can live like mad

of heritage planned (and planted by Mother Nature and Father Time). Some on the earth plane might preach our birth was somehow sinful or an accident, but such is not the case. We were planned by the highest and greatest and fiercest of forces. We might not see who we truly are on the surface, but every human matters—not just a saintly few who claim to be closest to God.

> **Sometimes you don't see the miracle because the miracle is you.**

Your physical life is meaningful and valuable, even if you just sit there. You are one of the creators. You, along with your ancestral body of relatives, coordinated your life in conjunction with the lives of those around you, and all of life springs outward from there. You might not be aware of your life's purpose and the details that go into that, but the pieces of the puzzle will eventually fit together, and the grand scheme of things shall be presented. We, given our limited perspectives, might not grasp the value of our own life, and there is a possibility that some of us might never be told all of the truth about our value. However, every step we take is sacred, even if we believe we are taking steps backward. We will reach our destination whether or not we believe in it, or ourselves, or the greater oneness of all there is: God, itself. We will reach the destination planned by the unmanifested Source. It is not a matter of if, it is a matter of when. The question is, how are we going to walk the journey?

We, earthlings, have two choices. We can walk it veiled from our worth, or we can walk in awareness. How will you walk? That is the question. Whatever you decide, you are loved. Loved by an endless ancestral family that knows no boundaries.

From an expansive point of view—one that spans time and space (including life between lives), our ancestral family wanted us so much—desperately wanted us in the picture—desperately wanted to acknowledge us and to be acknowledged. The problem is that humankind is unwilling to see beyond the surface at times. Sometimes fear and doubt are the enemies. It is fear and doubt that reject our bloodlines, ousts them from the conversation, and made-up stories about them. And the rest of the parishioners believed these stories as if they needed for us to be someone we didn't want to be. Our ancestors had the same problem when they walked the earth. Proselytizers insisted that our people were worthless, sinful creatures! It is our time to defend this from happening to future generations. It's our time now.

When you stand for humankind, proselytizers might hate you for it. They might blame you. They might accuse you of wrongdoing. They might do everything in their power to prove you wrong and reduce you down to someone you are not to make them look good, to fluff up their feathers, to prove that their way is the right way, to prove that they are right and righteous. Those against humanity wish for us to be afraid. When we are afraid and filled with shame, there is a tendency to stay nonchalant and less likely to begin toward our right back to self.

Few had the guts to stand on behalf of our ancestors! Communication lines were cut and severed, ancestors were abandoned, excluded from the dialogue. They want you to know that you are loved. Deeply loved. Loved so much that there is nothing you could do to break this love. They can see you for who you truly are. What if we weren't born in sin?

What if we belong to something vast and spectacular? What if we come from the stars? What if each of us is the missing link in our own lives—and the lives to those before us? What if our ancestors are proud of us? And they were proud of who they were during their own lives centuries past? They fought the good fight for our existence, and they did good. Yes, today, many modern conveniences distract us from identifying and recognizing the miraculous and capable tribe from which we are descendants.

Imagine that your ancestors want you to know that there is more to you than meets the eye. Your ancestors hold you in high regard. They love you. You are their prodigal son/daughter. They are impatiently waiting for your return,

where to find peace so you can live like mad

for the great family reunion. Your ancestors are on your side—always on your side. Whatever you decide to do, your ancestors support you one hundred percent. They truly believe in you; they trust that you will be kind and empathetic to all people.

All humans originate from the stars and we have the universe within us. We were planned (and planted) by something larger and grander than ever imagined. We were planned with all of us in mind—the human tribe. The oneness of human nature.

At the very least, we were planned by the stars. (What could be better than that?)

Interactive Element: Sacred Energy Life Force Genealogy Tree

Activity: Create a spiritual genealogy tree. Imagine your ancestral soul roots and acknowledge your connection that provide a sense of belonging and purpose. Write a short story on how recognizing these sacred soul connections brings you a sense of spiritual solidarity.

Example: "I am creating a soul tree and imagining that my great-grandmother was a healer in her village. This connection makes me feel proud and deeply rooted in my family's history. I now understand that my passion for holistic healing is part of my heritage, and this brings me a sense of belonging and purpose."

IN THE BEGINNING WAS THE "WORD"

"Sticks and stones will break my bones, but words will never hurt me!"

Remember that ol' schoolyard chant? Actually, it's a lie. Yes, sticks and stones can break bones, but words are also capable of hurting humanity. In fact, words can break the spirit of a person if we allow them too. Words have been used since the inception of the human language to build up, control, and tear down individuals, clans, communities, and even entire countries. Have you ever been reduced to a label or name-called something you weren't? This can have a big impact on our self-worth.

I will always remember the book *The Hidden Messages Of Water* by New York Times bestselling and internationally renowned scientist, Masaru Emoto (July 22, 1943 - October 17, 2014). In 1992, Dr. Emoto introduced the concept of water micro-clustering and magnetic resonance analysis technology. This is where his study on the true nature of water began. He realized that "the snowflake state revealed the individual face of each water drop." The doctor's scientific and high-speed photographic experiments captured the structure of water at the moment of freezing, exhibiting how thoughts, words, and feelings impact the blueprint molecules of water. His lab work demonstrated how words are profoundly influential and can be manifested and even obviously seen on a large scale, "frozen in time".

where to find peace so you can live like mad

Initially, Dr. Emoto placed a single drop of water into 50 Petri dishes and set them into a freezer for three hours at -13 °F. He observed the water crystal using a metal optical microscope with an external camera (Olympus BX60) at a magnification of 100 to 200 in a laboratory kept at 23 °F.

Due to the warming effect of light, the snowflake's lifespan could only be kept for two minutes. He focused light from the microscope onto the tip of the ice and observed through the external camera. Depending on the word attached to the Petri dish, the water crystal would either transform into a shiny hexagonal snowflake crystal or what appeared to oblong blobs. Depending on whether the water was from a natural spring or a kitchen tap, each drop reacted to and stored its experience, and this experience could be seen by the crystal formation. Doctor Emoto was able to manifest beautiful crystals from the waters of rivers and lakes. The crystal formed completely sourced from nature.

His findings provided the material for several books showcasing groundbreaking results. From his experiments, Dr. Emoto noticed that when optimistic words such as "truth" and "harmony" were directed towards water sources, the water droplets crystallized into well-formed snowflakes.

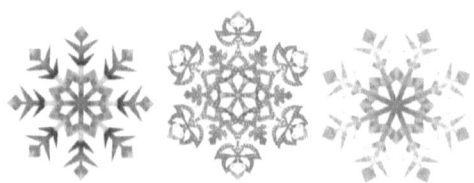

In contrast, when destructive words like "stupid" or "idiot" were attached to the Petri dishes holding the water, the molecules of water converted to dull and deformed broken shapes or blobs.

GOING BACK TO ZEN

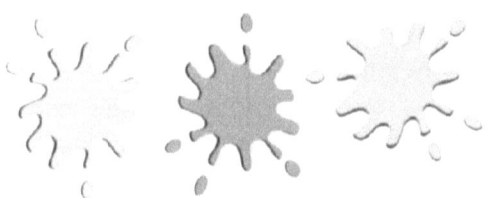

Since humans consist of seventy percent water, the results illustrated to the doctor how the thoughts and words humans direct at ourselves and others have a profound impact on our well-being. If we want peace for this planet and for ourselves, Dr. Emoto's revolutionary work provided further evidence of the power of words.

When we can see the evidence of how words can influence and morph water into crystallized works of art, then we become empowered. The thoughts we hold about ourselves shape who we are at a DNA level, and this influences how we feel about ourselves.

There may be times when we are given everything we could possibly think of and wish for, but if we do not hold kind thoughts for ourselves and others, well, we might feel down and out and wonder why happiness is so elusive. Since, as some might say, we live in "the best nation on earth" based on outside appearances, we might chastise ourselves for feeling bad when we "should be grateful." The truth is if someone (society, or even self) verbally attacks and puts us down, then, yes, we will feel bad. Imagine being called "anti-God" just because we do not fully agree with someone else's religious beliefs. What is the solution? Listen to the dialogue. Have we been put down by others? Are we repeating the same attitude and words in our own internal dialogue? Or are we kind to ourselves and others? Whichever the way, we will feel the aftermath.

Recovery from suffering might take several trials and errors, or it can be instant. I've felt the repercussions in my own life. Words I have used to describe myself can help or hinder me. Dr. Emoto's water experiments provided evidence to at least be cognizant of my inner dialogue and the words I

where to find peace so you can live like mad

use to describe myself. By monitoring my inner dialogue, I am able to recognize when I'm not being nice to myself or when I am criticizing myself unnecessarily.

The words I use to describe myself can be a natural healing remedy. Words influence our attitude and behavior. I notice that a mere word we use to describe ourselves can hurt and divide and pull us down, or they can inspire motivation and prompt lifelong purpose.

> "The moment you change your perception is the moment you rewrite the chemistry of your body." --Bruce Lipton

Each word carries energy. Based on traditional medicine and ancient healing modalities, even one word can remedy discomforts, physical ailments, and suffering. I am an active participant and in direct control of the healing process. Healing with words is based on the premise that "first there was the word." Words form assumptions, and assumptions are powerful, whether intended or not intended. Thoughts can determine my mood, motivation, and inspiration. Words can add fuel to the fire or extinguish the fire (and the desire) completely. Words determine attitudes and behaviors. Imagine how different it would be if we assumed everyone is our friend versus everyone is our enemy. (Ever notice the verbiage used in politics that describe people as aliens and foreigners instead of humans and neighbors?) The way we treat the person changes drastically. Imagine if we assumed we were born in sacredness instead of sin. It could possibly make all the difference in the world. Just in the body, we could relax instead of holding and carrying around tension.

Imagination and belief can be an especially useful solution when maintaining and improving my health. The energy words can generate a subtle and, at times, potent modality, which serves as an additional healing component to self-recovery or a sabotaging element.

Whereas Western medicine details and addresses each specific part of the body, Eastern medicine diagnoses the body as one unit, and it is understood as a mini-universe consisting of a multi-faceted mind, body, emotions, and spirit found within the human energy system.

Interactive Element: Words of Power

Activity: Write down ten positive affirmations or words that describe you. Meditate on each word for a minute, focusing on the feelings it evokes. Pay attention to the changes in mood or perspective after the exercise.

Example: "Today, I wrote down the words 'resilient,' 'kind,' and 'capable.' Meditating on 'resilient' made me feel strong and unwavering. Repeating 'kind' filled my heart with warmth, and 'capable' boosted my confidence. I felt a wave of positivity wash over me, setting a serene tone for my day."

Words are much more vital to our physical, emotional, and spiritual health and harmony than typically given credit. Humans are inventive beings. Our purpose is to create in some way. words are essential to feelings of fulfillment and expansion. they are the spark that ignites us to leave something of ourselves behind. The aftermath of our words have the power to become our legacy.

WORDS ARE ENERGY

We, humans, are energetic beings. Our organs, tissues, and even diseases are made of energy. Everything is made of energy, and everything around us is moving energy. New physics reveals that our thoughts and emotions are energy as well. Emotional stresses are at first thoughts that transform into malleable vibrations stored in various parts of our body, affecting organs, muscle tissue, and body systems. A disease is a fluctuating ball of condensed energy. All people, physical things, emotions, attitudes, conversations, and relationships create a vibration. When we want something, the body moves in a way that makes this happen. For instance, I wanted the truth about the history of adoption. For more than twenty years, my body got up every morning to study, research, and investigate. I wasn't able to put it to rest until the truth emerged before me. Whereas thoughts that separate humanity attract additional ideas of division, this also means that unifying thoughts generate harmonizing and peaceful spaces. (I like to refer to peace as PEACE: People Enjoying A Cohesive Environment). Being informed of the mind and body link and the inherent authority of thoughts and words (or the power of thoughtful words) places us in control of our health and can serve as preventative medicine. Preventative medicine is the most effective of treatments.

where to find peace so you can live like mad

> The difference between the right word and the almost right word is the difference between lightning and a lightning bug.
>
> ~Mark Twain

For the benefit of the whole being, both instinct and logic need to be acknowledged for all components to work in conjunction with each other, and thus in harmony. Using words to give ourselves an identity is not meant to replace the prescriptions of a medical professional, and it is not always a blatant remedy—although some have experienced the use of words to be effective immediately. Recovery from severe emotional pain depends on additional factors, such as whether or not we have specific sabotaging thoughts still confined somewhere in the body that may be contributing to our frame of reference.

Dr. Bruce H. Lipton, a biologist, published in the late 1990s the groundbreaking book, Biology Of Belief: Unleashing The Power Of Consciousness, Matter, and Miracles, which shaped scientific perception and served as a stepping stone towards discovering the power of thoughts and words. He introduced the field of "new biology" through research between the interaction of the mind and body. Dr. Lipton's work demonstrated the union between perception and the chemistry of the body, affirming the idea that outside signals can control our health and well-being.

Using the power of the mind-body-emotion-soul connection, we can communicate with our cells, our body parts, our organs, and even send goodwill messages for them using the language of imagination and energy.

Without the awareness of the mind's capacity to shape the cellular make-up, illness can rest dormant and manifest into the development of such things like addictions or bad habits triggered by individual thoughts and beliefs. When focused on inabilities, we tend to grieve. Alternatively, when we pay attention to our abilities, our mood shifts. We find a way to get the job done, and we are motivated to do more—even whatever it takes to accomplish tasks, or reach a goal. A mere shift in identity can uplift our disposition, strengthen, and empower us.

Emotions are...

...energy in motion.

Humans tend to mask (or try to hide from) tender emotions because we do not want to suffer. But we do suffer if we do not take the time to appreciate ourselves or pay attention to our value. Emotions like depression, anxiety, fear, sleeplessness, shame, or guilt can eventually lead to physical pain unless we give them immediate attention and see ourselves for who we truly are—the whole self. That is when we can stop and take notice and then deconstruct any limiting words we use to describe ourselves, sabotaging thoughts, or a misconstrued belief system. Beneath the surface, you are genuine, joy, light, peace, truth, innocence, love (and nothing less).

Single words can build a divisive empire. I've seen how the word orphan has been expanded to include children of single or "poor" parents and thus used to build a global empire and a following. I've observed up close and personal how entire families and tribes can be ignored and ousted as if they do not exist just because a child is labeled an "orphan" and adopted. In my own life, being called an adoptee has minimized my human right to know and have access to my biological family, as if such loss has little value.

where to find peace so you can live like mad

One word can make all the difference in the world.

 Because of my "orphan" status (according to a typed up document), there was little reason to look for what was presumed to be non-existent family members. However, once international (and domestic) adoptees realized that every single human comes from a human family, and evidence of families started appearing from afar for countless adoptees, we suddenly had grounds to look for relatives. I am motivated to find the missing pieces in my life—missing pieces, which could be the cause of any feelings of internal grieving or grief that might have been felt at a low-grade level. Perhaps some of us who have been removed from our family tribes are feeling the consequences of this loss within our own energetic system, which lead us to feelings of subtle, yet nagging angst, and consequently manifests in one way or another. And because some of us were led to believe that we were orphaned, we are less likely to search. Thus we go through life unfulfilled. Some of us just can't pinpoint where this "something is missing" feeling comes from, so there could be a tendency to deny or ignore it.
 When I shifted my identity from that of an orphan (and even an adoptee) to someone who was born to a real expansive family (like all humans are), I am brought closer to oneness and wholeness and the reunion with my tribe. The shift in identity can change everything. When we enlarge who we are, we empower ourselves to access ethnic and cultural rights, and we are compelled to move toward a personal revolution. This shift in dynamic speaks volumes against a lucrative industry, which labels children as orphans or calls them needy or special needs and exploits families in order to process children for the overseas adoption market.

GOING BACK TO ZEN

> When the thoughts are changed, the mind is changed, when the mind is changed, the man is changed, when the man is changed, the society is changed, when the society is changed, the nation is changed, and when the nations change for the better, we say there is plenty and prosperity all over the world!
>
> --Mahatma Gandhi

The human is a package of pulsating power constantly engaged with a plethora of energy. We are not separate from our environment. Our thoughts may be central in shaping our interconnected world. Therefore, we can prevent disease, and we can create health and well-being. The great miracle about this? What's the best part? The words we decide to use to describe ourselves are all free, and they have lasting profound effects that can last for generations.

If your parents (or anyone around you) have ever called you words like, guilty, a thief, a liar, lazy, distrustful, a bum, unworthy up to no good, or if you have ever called yourself sick or weak or unsafe, or if you have ever been accused of being bossy, having an infatuation with blood ties, patriarchal, hit the refresh button and call yourself the exact opposite for the day: genuine, honest, giving, truthful, energized, trustworthy, worthwhile, healthy, smart, strong, interested and interesting, fair, modest

I bet you will feel a whole lot better. When you feel better, you are aligned with the truth of who you are: Your where to find peace so you can live like mad true, innate, and authentic self. There is more goodness in you than you could ever imagine.

Interactive Element: Energy Mapping

Activity: Draw a body outline and mark where you feel tension or discomfort. Next to each spot, write down any negative words or thoughts you associate with that area. Replace them with positive affirmations and visualize the tension melting away as you repeat these affirmations.

Example: "I drew a body outline and marked tension in my shoulders and neck. Next to these areas, I wrote 'stress' and 'burdened.' Replacing these words with 'relaxed' and 'supported' and visualizing the tension melting away left me feeling lighter and more at ease."

WHEN THEY ACCUSE YOU OF BEING "BAD"

As a child, I was led to believe that humans are sinful in nature or born "bad" and at risk of being sent to hell if we didn't abide by certain church rules, kind of like an everlasting jail card. This had a profound impact on me. During church sermons, I would often wonder what it would be like to burn forever in fiery red hot flames. Today, after studying eastern philosophy, I believe that humans are sacred in nature. To think any less of ourselves and others can be detrimental to our well-being and even sabotage our health and relationships. No one likes to be falsely judged or accused. I'm sure all humans have been falsely accused at least once in their life—including you. When authorities assume that we are sinful in nature and thus in need to change in order to win their approval or welcomed into their group or even into heaven, this can cause us to be a little resentful. When we are taught that humans are born sinful, then it is easier to judge, stigmatize, and treat them as if bad people. That type of assumption tends to cause more division and separation. Humanity tends not to give as much consideration or practice as much compassion. To acknowledge the sacredness within all people can change our perception of humanity, and especially if that person is in touch with their innate nature, that perception is mirrored back at us. We are better able to see the value of every person. When we treat others with consideration, it tends to be returned.

where to find peace so you can live like mad

Placing value on diverse thoughts prompts respect and admiration for each individual's ability to survive on this difficult earthly terrain. Also, we can be proud of "self" and others for the accomplishments all have made despite challenges. From this place of acknowledgment, we find solutions at the core roots.

A great many of us contend with some form of discrimination, verbal harassment, and misconstrued attitudes against our character. It doesn't matter who we are or our background. These misconceptions add up and can plague us, which can hurt our self-esteem and confidence even into our elder years. Remnants of hurtful comments can influence generations after us. If we did not receive nurturing and defense as children, we have a lot of catching up to do. We must not only "love self," but we also need to find the reason to like ourselves and talk to ourselves in the most sensitive and protective way possible. Sometimes we need to write down a list of amazing things about ourselves to serve as a gentle reminder. This attention aligns the ego with the authentic self. If we are not aware of the need to love and like the self, any emotional pain can eventually snowball into physical pain.

> "Everything you will ever need to know is within you; the secrets of the universe are imprinted on the cells of your body."   ~Dan Millman

We must like the "unlikable" parts of "self" and not allow perceived faults block us from seeing the true self dormant under the surface. How do we treat others when we like them? What are we willing to do for them? Typically we put extra effort into the relationship. (I've found that we must give ourselves the same consideration.) When feeling down, it's time to pay a little more attention to yourself and accept the unacceptable parts, the so-called unlovable part. Don't just be yourself; I believe what can help more is to like yourself—especially the parts deemed unlikable by others. Acceptance of the "imperfections" can be transforming. A belief in capabilities and potential can result because it is human nature to work for things we believe in. The proactive human spirit is ready and willing to stand one's ground, to nurture, protect, and defend oneself and others for the benefit of all of humanity.

Whatever therapeutic words we decide to use, we will notice the body slightly changing, following whatever the mind believes to be true. Endorphins are released in the brain, and a natural high occurs. Sometimes the cure arrives as gentle as an uplift in one's mood, but this can change everything! A good mood can serve to motivate one to move the body or to work on another project—and finish it! We are energized and ready for more. At the end of the day, we are glad we went ahead and took action!

Whatever we do, we must like ourselves as we go about our business, and suddenly we feel relaxed and strengthened. Give yourself a thumbs up! (Just don't do this in public or they'll think you're mad! ;-)) Acceptance of all that is allows for the chips to fall as they may; we remain calm and carry on, secure in who we are and our ability to survive and thrive because we know we are rooted in the tribal strength of who we really are: truth and love.

The advice to feel our feelings in order to heal used to bother me. In fact, it was a pet peeve of mine during my twenties. I wanted to know why. No one could give me a good reason, so I read a ton of books trying to find the answer. I used to assume that the modern-day psychologists advocated for people to drown themselves in their own sad stories and pity parties. What good is it to continuously feel feelings, I wondered. Doesn't this motivate us to wallow in our pain?

Emotional pain, blame, and shame lies in the heart of just about every condition. Many of us assume that we had a decent life, and no recovery is needed, but still almost everyone has had at least one insult (even if unintentional) or more hurled at them that can live on in the body and deplete us of our energy. Even seemingly trivial words can have profound effects, depending on our perception of the word and the intention of the person using it. Every word carries energy. It is easy to believe that we're "not good enough" or "not like someone else" or that someone else should do this or that. We might not want to change certain dogmatic beliefs we've been taught to believe as children due to an innate fear of the unknown. A solution exists. I've found that trusting myself and my life plan (even if I don't know what it is) can calm nerves, help me to relax, and guide me into believing in the tenacity of the human spirit. Trust in the sacred energy life force that is within each, and every one of us offers strength during the darkest moments. Trust yourself!

Sometimes the key is just one sentence: "It's not your fault." Or replacing the dogma that we, humans, are sinful in nature, with the notion that "we are truly sacred in nature," a belief based on ancient and traditional Asian philosophies that date back thousands of years. And to access our sacredness, we revert to the body's energy system for balance and harmonize with our real sacred self. Reiki, meditations, yoga, tai chi, martial arts, Qigong, guided visualization, diaphragmatic (controlled) breathing techniques, and other complementary therapies operate from the premise that all of life (and the afterlife) is energy.

The consciousness of our sacred origin is the cure. Awareness of our innate healing power provides us with the key. Sensations of insightfulness, lightbulb moments, peace, joy, contentment, relaxation, and understanding are all tools that can be used to alleviate burdensome emotions derived from our own personal resource box.

Easing suffering can be as simple as changing the way one thinks about "self," which evolves into less stress and leads to inner strength. One's health can also be a discovery into a harmful relationship or lead a person to be aware of certain thoughts that might trigger one to grab that alcoholic drink or to pull out a cigarette. Sometimes self-love, like, and pride can alter one's reality immediately; other times, it is a process. Belief in one's own value and imagination are innate and limitless tools that can minister one's ability to meet and defeat heavy habitual emotions. Sooner or later, we need to feel the feelings of loss, grief, sorrow, anxiety, anger, rage, to push the pent up energy out of our system.

> **EMPATHY,**
> **COMPASSION, AND LOVE**
> toward ourselves and
> others, the formula for an
> elevated and harmonious
> life flow, and peace.
> Visualize unconditional love
> (& like) for self, family,
> community, and humanity.

What are you feeling? Sadness? Rage? Grief? Fears? I use these heavy emotions to motivate myself into exploration and then action. I eventually diagnose the source of the issue and then find the right self-care solution for myself. My dad has imagined throwing his grief into a large public garbage dump as we drive by. I sometimes imagine seeing discouraging emotions as clouds and physically clearing them out with my hands. Whenever we feel heaviness, we can collect the energy with our imaginations, and disperse the excess out to the universe or into the ground as if playing with clouds for a little bit. Imagination is a free resource we can rely on—a tool we can utilize whenever need be. Feel the heavy emotions of the past. Now visualize directing them out of your body's energy system. Hit the refresh button: Imagine as the light fills and replenishes you.

Element: Self-Compassion Journal

Activity: Keep a daily journal where you write down instances where you felt judged or accused. Counter each negative experience with three positive attributes about yourself. Reflect on how these positive affirmations impact your self-perception over time.

Example: "Today, I was criticized at work for a mistake I made. In my journal, I wrote about the incident and then listed three positive attributes: 'hardworking,' 'dedicated,' and 'quick learner.' Reflecting on these qualities helped me regain my value and see the mistake as a learning opportunity."

LOVE IS G.O.D

The body is not only made up of isolated parts to be fixed but an amazing web of intricate detail. To truly return to health, each layer of our being needs to be acknowledged. Self-love and care strengthen the immune system, harmonize the function of glands and organs, and push pains outward as a result. Pure energy opens the blocked channels, the meridians, and balances the chakras. When self-love and care are given freely and regularly, toxins dissipate from the body. As demonstrated by the water droplets that transform into striking crystallized formations seen as snowflakes on Petri dishes, health and well-being can be maintained because of kind and encouraging words. Self-kindness generates stress reduction, relaxation, and the strengthening and maintenance of the immune system. Love and kindness directed at oneself can help us to heal. When permitting ourselves to align with the wisdom of our ancestors, energy blockages and suppressed emotions are released, and we are better able to achieve goals and see from an empowered outlook. Miraculous answers come into view. It is easier for us to overcome obstacles because we have made a commitment to the true self. (I imagine that our ancestors appreciate this.)

Among the numerous harmonizing medicinal options to choose from today, we find that aligning ourselves with our core root is a gentle holistic healing method that validates the right to freedom from dogma and soothes on many levels: physical, mental, emotional and spiritual. Reverting to ancient healing techniques has become increasingly acceptable around the world, especially since science has verified the existence of universal life energy. Sacred life force permeates our entire being and all living things. Like air, it circulates throughout and around the body. When we align with our core roots, we align with the true self.

God is Love = Love is God

The harmonious flow of life force results in a stronger immune system. It is the way of nature. Unhealthy patterns, misconstrued emotions, and imbalances interrupt this flow and lead to illness. Subtle energy is responsible for our body's processes at every level. Awareness and openness to include all of the self—even the part of ourselves that seems undesirable—is a form of self-care which balances and restores the body's stream of energy, steering us to walk the path of the person we were born to be.

This self-respect, as a bonus, enables us to attune with the more genuine part of the self. Trusting the universal plan set forth by our greater and deeply connected selves pushes out fear, doubt, and misunderstandings. Meditation (or listening for God, as some might say) can be used to increase intuition and promote limitless benefits of spiritual connection. Ancient healing based on natural remedies is gentle and subtle, which makes for an empowering arena available for anyone. Trusting ourselves does not require anything but receptiveness and the belief that anything is possible. The benefits are mysterious.

For two thousand years, proselytizers refused to allow the natives to practice natural healing methods that belonged to the earth and their culture. This ethnic and ancestral persecution still influences humanity today. We as humans have been shamed for so-called uncivilized traditions, and accusations have gravely altered our perception of self and our self-esteem. Because we are merely humans, the sacredness of who we are has been ignored and dismissed and vilified. It was not uncommon for missionaries to associate the practice of Traditional Chinese Medicine and Ayurveda, the traditional Hindu system of medicine, as evil and even claimed native cultures to be the work of a devil. Some tried to oust and outlaw the ancient practices from its native soil.

LOVE IS G.O.D.

To acknowledge that our ancestors believed in the same universal power as the missionaries can empower us. This means that God is also on our side. Unknown to the proselytizers, the locals believed in the power of Mother Earth's resources—the same source as God—the same source from which all of life originates. Taoists refer to the Source as the unmanifested. The natives regard and utilize the divine from a different angle. The power to heal came from natural resources accessible to everyone and anyone.

God =

Goodness over Dogma

To establish a lasting effect, we have the opportunity to deny or accept the movement of sacred life force energy. This means we are active participants in the healing process and totally in control of our destiny. The alignment with the true self is noninvasive and does not rely on any organized religion at all. Connecting with our authentic, ethical self is merely a natural remedy. There is no particular dogma that the individual must learn to be touched by its energy. One must only be open to the possibilities. Today's alternative and complementary medicines have already been proven effective to cure people through all walks of life in the eastern

where to find peace so you can live like mad

world. When attempting to uplift oneself, consideration for self and others unlocks the door to many fascinating ideas and philosophies, which can lead us back to ourselves.

Interactive Element: Acts of Kindness

Activity: Perform three acts of kindness this week, either for yourself or others. Document these acts and reflect on how they influence your sense of peace and connection with the world around you.

Example: "I helped an elderly neighbor with her groceries, smiled at a stranger, and wrote a heartfelt note to a friend. Each act of kindness made me feel more connected and filled my heart with joy. It reminded me that simple gestures can create a peaceful and loving community."

UNPLUGGING & BREAKING FREE

In today's digital age, social media can feel like an inescapable part of life. It connects us, entertains us, and informs us. However, for many, it can also be a source of stress, anxiety, and even bullying. I know this all too well. After being bullied on social media, I found myself dreading each notification and avoiding my accounts altogether. This experience was a key motivator for writing this book, and I want to share with you how I successfully disconnected from social media and found peace.

Tips to Recover from Social Media Stress

1. Set Boundaries: Limit your social media usage to specific times of the day. Use apps that track and limit your screen time.

2. Curate Your Feed: Unfollow or mute accounts that cause stress or negativity. Follow pages and people who inspire and uplift you.

3. Digital Detox: Take regular breaks from social media. Start with a day, then a weekend, and gradually extend to longer periods. Or go ahead and disconnect completely if you feel the need.

where to find peace so you can live like mad

4. Engage in Offline Activities: Rediscover hobbies and activities you enjoy that don't involve a screen. Reading, hiking, painting, and cooking are great alternatives.

5. Connect in Real Life: Spend more time with friends and family in person. Build relationships that aren't based on likes and comments.

6. Mindfulness Practices: Incorporate meditation, yoga, and breathing exercises into your routine to help manage anxiety and stress.

7. Seek Support: If social media bullying has affected your mental health, consider talking to a therapist or counselor.

Interactive Element: Social Media Detox Plan

Activity: Create a Personalized Social Media Detox Plan

Step 1: Write down your current social media habits and identify the main sources of stress.

Step 2: Set clear boundaries for social media use, such as specific times and durations for checking accounts.

Step 3: Plan offline activities to replace social media time. List at least three hobbies or interests you'd like to explore.

Step 4: Unfollow or mute any accounts that contribute to negativity. Follow new accounts that promote positivity and inspiration.

Step 5: Schedule regular digital detoxes. Start with a one-day detox and gradually extend it.

Step 6: Journal your experiences during the detox periods, noting any changes in mood and well-being.

Example: "I started my social media detox by unfollowing accounts that caused me stress and following pages about nature and wellness. I set a rule to check my accounts only twice a day for ten minutes each. During my first weekend detox, I rediscovered my love for painting and took a long hike. These activities brought me a sense of peace and fulfillment that social media never could. By the end of the weekend, I felt more connected to myself and less anxious."

THE PAIN MIGHT NOT BE IN YOUR HEAD

Ever complained to a friend, family member, or foe about something painful only to be met by a dismissive comment like, "the pain is just in your head"? ...Well, I'm here to say the pain might not be in your head, it might be in your body! According to eastern philosophy, biology reflects the harmony of the human body in accordance with its environment. Our biology influences our biography, and our biography influences our biology. This idea is reflected in the full circle of Taoism encompassing the yin and the yang. If the body lacks essential minerals, our mood is influenced. When the mood is down, the view of the world can be painfully tainted, and dejection inhibits self-care. Fortunately, Mother Earth provides all that we need to nourish ourselves.

Humans are bombarded with daily strain, environmental pressures, and overloaded with non-stop data that hits us from every direction, and every moment of our waking and sleeping state. This, of course, has been recently due to living in the digital information age and compounded with the current coronavirus culture. Because of the convenience of cell phones, we can tuck away massive bits of data around our wrists, in our pockets, wherever we sit, and even under the pillow! The surplus of information has never occurred before in human history. We are being bombarded with messages, even while sleeping. Don't blame yourself if you're feeling overwhelmed and on guard!

GOING BACK TO ZEN

Tension can be felt when humans resist particular events. It is the body's strategy to rise to the challenge and confront life-threatening scenarios armed with heightened alertness, focus, additional strength, and stamina. The emergencies that provoke tension are called stressors, and they are ignited by a whole range of situations, from blatant physical danger to making a presentation, to meeting a deadline.

Most stress comes from things like being burdened with work, incompatible priorities, unplanned events, interpersonal relationships, unpleasant scenarios, pushing, pressure and prodding from others, and so on. Not only do stressors impact our lifestyle as we exert effort to handle them, but they can also elicit a great deal of emotional suffering.

I have recently learned, after noticing the weakness in my body, that the human body needs a certain amount of minerals every day to function at its best. Problems can arise when our diet does not supply our bodies with essential nutrients. Being deficient can greatly damper performance as well as the body's overall health. Although I tried to eat a healthy diet and drank mostly water throughout my adult life, I suddenly started feeling a deep level of chronic muscle pain and joint inflammation throughout my body. When I noticed that I would become sleepy after I drank a large amount of soda, I limited consumption and started drinking more water. I was comparing myself against my dad, who drank vitamin water and rarely (if ever) complained of body pain even into his eighties. He showed better health than me. Because of my concern, I relented to the idea of living out the rest of my life with persistent pain, but the thought caused me to be exhausted and anxious, and my concentration (or my confidence) seemed to decline.

I also coped with chronic muscle pain, leg/foot cramps, and twitches under my right eye, but I didn't want to go to a medical doctor—at least not just yet. I wanted to study the cause of my ailments. After researching my symptoms, I learned I lacked various nutrients, one mineral in particular: magnesium. It turns out my chronic muscle pain and joint inflammation had to do with a lack of minerals.

where to find peace so you can live like mad

A well-balanced diet can supply the body with the support it needs to prevent body imbalances and thus nourish the brain. The symptoms of nutrient deficiency present themselves when undernourishment is at an advanced level. The pain wasn't in my head! The pain had to do with my body's lack of vitamins and minerals. If we do not feel fully our best, it could be due to being depleted of foundational nutrients—and not caused by diabetes, cancer, or worse case scenarios that plague the mind when body pains suddenly show up. (For those of us who are not permitted to access our family's ancestry due to draconian adoption laws, preventative medicine is one way to care for self.) I began to take a daily magnesium supplement, and within only a week, I felt an improvement. Since then, my muscle and joint pain, inflammation, and leg cramps decreased. Being relieved of pain definitely improved my mood! I could study and write better too!

Just a little reminder:

MINERALS AND VITAMINS
Foundational MicroNutrients:

MINERALS:
Inorganic Hold onto their chemical structure Soil and water, chemically simpler Not all are needed Chemical elements Indestructible

VITAMINS:
Organic Can be broken down by heat, air, and acid From plants and animals All vitamins are needed Easily destroyed when cooked Chemical compounds Destructible

I am not a medical doctor, but I suggest that if you are feeling soreness or achiness, make sure to nourish and protect your body with minerals. Maybe visit a naturopathic doctor to get started or consult with your medical doctor in addition with your innate wisdom and research. I started to pay attention to my vitamin and mineral supplements when I felt muscle achiness. Magnesium consists of more than 300 enzyme systems that regulate biochemical reactions like muscle and nerve function, blood glucose control that is required for energy production. A healthy dose of magnesium calms the mood, dampens muscle inflammation, relaxes blood vessels, and decreases blood pressure.

The take away for me has been to consider the free or at least less expensive, less invasive, and less radical remedies first, which is found and easily attainable in inexpensive resources. For the body to stay strong and energized, look into essential minerals. If we do not have fresh greens immediately available, it's never too late to start taking a supplement, at least if that makes sense for you. As the Buddhists advocate, everything in moderation.

Due to the instant mind and muscle improvement after taking magnesium, I often wonder what miracle we could have experienced if we had been immediately informed about its value after Dad's injury in 1984. Of course, we cannot go back steeped in wishful thinking. We can only go onward and forward from where we are. If you ever feel sluggish, follow your own sense of direction, check in with a naturopath and/or a medical doctor (whichever makes you the most comfortable) before starting anything new or making drastic changes.

Foundational care is fundamental when it comes to achieving a clarified state of mind. If your body hurts, add encouraging and uplifting self-talk to your daily schedule. Body pain can sabotage us from focusing, which in turn distracts us from being able to write. Even the most pristine among us can forget to be kind to the body! If you are in pain or stressed, make sure your body has the resources it needs to work at its optimum. This could be the missing link. (In the next chapter I mention another one of my missing links.)

Interactive Element: Body Awareness Meditation

Activity: Engage in a guided body scan meditation focusing on identifying and acknowledging pain. Journal about any insights or connections you discover regarding how emotional states affect physical sensations. Talk with your body. Ask what are you supposed to learn from the pain?

Example: "During the body scan meditation, I noticed a persistent ache in my lower back. I reflected on how this pain could be linked to stress at work. By acknowledging the pain and sending it love and healing energy, I felt a significant reduction in discomfort and a sense of inner peace."

CLEAN WATER and FRESH PRODUCE: More of the population is realizing the dominant result of a balanced diet on our physical, emotional, mental, and spiritual health. A pure diet can generate greater health, upbeat emotional states, a clearer mind and performance, and increased alignment with our individual truths. Drinking fresh water and food oxygenates and feeds the brain.

ESSENTIALS FROM MOTHER NATURE

    I recently reinvestigated the way food is treated as medicine in Asia and learned how crucial it is for the human body to absorb a daily amount of vitamins to function at its optimum level and, more importantly, less painfully. Making sure that I at least take a supplement is now as important to me as silent time. While meditation helps me to access my true self, minerals and vitamins serve as an essential foundation for my stability. Used together, my frame of reference has improved and expanded.
    If we do not feed the body enough of the essentials it needs to function, we might experience physical pain. Physical pain influences our mood. This pain could signal us to treat ourselves and others differently; we might even place unnecessary blame upon ourselves or others. The nutrients from the earth are vital and serve as preventative medicine.
    In the busy world of modern society, it is increasingly difficult to farm our own organic fruits and vegetables. Add to that the convenience of fast food joints, Uber deliveries, frozen supermarket finds, and pre-packaged foods! Benefiting from fresh produce seems to be slipping away. It wasn't until I traveled to Vietnam that I fell in love with the idea of street-side vendors, fruit and veggie stands, lunch and soup carts, each offering a plethora of recently harvested produce from fruit trees and vegetable plants. All of that inspired me to explore fresh ingredients to experiment with new recipes, like soups, salads, and stir-fries. After that trip, I

appreciated the idea of playing with the natural ingredients that go into Vietnamese dishes. I climbed out of my comfort zone, and mother nature opened a limitless landscape for me to explore.

Vitamins are vital when it comes to keeping our heart healthy. Supplementing with fruits and vegetables is necessary to keep the heart working strong and long.

If you feel devoid of energy, you could be deprived of the daily dose of vitamins your body hungers for, and the solution could be at your fingertips. Although there are many vitamins, a certain amount of each one is necessary to keep the body healthy. There are several categorizations of vitamins, including A, B, C, D, and E. Each one serves a unique purpose.

Those of us who do not get enough of the vitamins A, B1, and B2 will feel tired, and a loss of appetite. Other symptoms include mental and emotional stress. Supplements that contain vitamins B6, B12, B17, D, E, and folic acid, are known to help the heart remain healthy, boost the immune system, energize, and even fight cancer.

The most common causes of vitamin and mineral deficiency include a poor diet, alcoholism, stress, or medications that interfere with the body's absorption of nutrients. If you notice that you lack in an area, do not try to catch up on what's been missing by taking more than needed. According to Taoism, the middle way leads to less emotional pain and even liberation.

The entire B family contributes to the well-being of the body. Scientists have isolated the vitamin into eight variants. As with other vitamin classes, a deficiency in the B vitamin can result in various conditions such as weight loss, weakness, stress, diarrhea, dementia, and anemia, among other things. Although other vitamins are essential to our diet, the Bs are among the most important. As a whole, the vitamin B lineage works on the health of the skin, a faster metabolism, and an overall better immune system. The B family can also ward against stress and depression. Don't forget to consider it when planning your healthcare protocol. When the body lacks B1 (thiamine to process carbohydrates), and B2 (riboflavin relieves sore throat, mouth sores, swollen tongue, bloodshot eyes, sensitivity to light), it feels tired, weak, or a loss of appetite. Other symptoms include mental and emotional stress or even anxiety. Among vitamins and supplements, one of the most common for energy is folic acid. Folic acid is a B vitamin that has been proven to increase energy levels. The vitamin known as NADH (B12) is often used to remedy chronic fatigue. Like I've mentioned, I am not a doctor, but I do try to listen to my body, and if I feel achiness, I look into my vitamin and mineral intake to take care of my foundational cellular health.

Vitamin C is known as an antioxidant, which prevents the damaging effects that cholesterol has on the body. Along with the prevention of cholesterol, it boosts vitamin E with its functions to improve overall heart health. A dosage of 400 international units of vitamin C and E are the recommended amount for most people. The heart is in need of consistent care. When we eat a proper diet and take the necessary vitamins, we are well on our way to keeping the heart strong. Vitamin E is essential to prevent cholesterol from harming the arteries that surround the heart. Anytime cholesterol oxidizes, it sticks to the sides of these vessels and can lead to blockages, which can pose problems. Research has shown Vitamin E can potentially prevent heart disease by opening up and protecting the arteries and eliminate obstructions.

Don't forget to get adequate amounts of calcium and vitamin D for strengthening your bones. The Journal of the American Geriatrics Society reported in February 2004 that elderly women who took a vitamin D supplement plus calcium for three months reduced their risk of falling by 49% compared with consuming calcium alone, according to researchers at the University of Basel in Switzerland. That same year, the magazine Neurology pointed out that women who take at least 400 IUs are 40% less likely to develop multiple sclerosis compared to those who do not. Also, of more than 3,000 veterans, those who consumed more than 645 international units each day of the vitamin (along with more than 4 grams of cereal fiber) had a 40% reduction of risk in the development of premalignant colon lesions. Remember

GOING BACK TO ZEN

Vitamin D for your defense against cancer cell growth. "It also stimulates your pancreas to make insulin," says Dr. Holick, Ph.D., MD, professor of medicine at the Boston University Medical Center. Another one of its many benefits include the regulation of the body's immune system.

Most doctors recommend foods that are naturally rich in vitamin E, such as almonds, hazel and pine nuts, sunflower seeds, and greens like swiss chard, spinach, and kale. Avocado, broccoli, papaya, and olives also contain the nutrient. Your doctor may suggest an additional E vitamin supplement if you do not have access to fresh produce or for individuals who have had a heart attack. Look for an all-organic supplement without fillers, or anti-caking agents.

Iron carries oxygen to the body's tissues. Not enough can leave you tired and weak and may even inhibit the performance of the brain.

The mineral Zinc is needed by every cell in the body. This mineral plays a crucial role in hundreds of processes in the human body, like supporting the immune system, joints, tissues, and aiding cell growth. The body is unable to produce zinc on its own, which is why we need to eat enough food that contains the mineral, drink enough water, and take the appropriate supplements that will give our cells the zinc they need. Also, zinc has been known to contribute to the ability to see, taste, smell, and the healing of wounds. Leg cramps could be a sign of not having enough zinc in the body. Zinc also fights the symptoms of a cold. Although zinc is an essential mineral, taking too much of it for over an extended period of time could damage the immune system.

Even though we may be following a healthy diet, we might not be getting all that we need. We can strive to find the right vitamins necessary in the event of an emergency situation or undernourishment. Being deficient in nutrients can damper performance as well as the overall health of the body. If you need a focused mind, these earthly essentials could be just what you are looking for. In my honest opinion, a multi-vitamin is sufficient, mixed in with as many garden greens as we can get our hands-on.

where to find peace so you can live like mad

FOUR EASY TEAS

I'm a big coffee drinker, but during my late twenties, a curiosity in teas emerged. At that time, I had no idea that there were any benefits at all. Come to find out that teas have many health-wise perks, including medicinal advantages! To be able to focus, reduce stress, and write effectively, I might make myself a cup of tea to boost my mood.

Ginger Tea
Ginger root has become one of my favorite treatments for whenever anyone in the family suspects we're feeling sick. At our house, we use a home-made flu and cold remedy combining grated ginger (keeping the skin on makes the concoction much spicier), freshly squeezed lime (or lemon), and honey into hot water stirred into a tea. We can also use these ingredients as soothing additions for soups and dishes.

When it comes to everyday ailments, ginger root has been a useful solution for us. The root offers many advantages, particularly for curing headaches, colds, and flu. One of the most common uses of ginger is to treat an upset stomach. If you don't have fresh ginger to grate, bottled ginger ale (even if flat) and crackers can assist an upset tummy. For the last few decades, civilizations such as from the Americas and Asia have used the root in cooking and as medicine to prevent ailments ranging from motion sickness to athlete's foot. The anti-inflammatory properties can also lessen the intensity of rheumatoid arthritis and cramp pain.

Whenever I suspect a cold or flu coming on, I'll look for a nub of ginger. (The longer the ginger remains in the ground before being harvested, the spicier it gets.) The crops, which are obtained roughly five months or so after being planted, can be used for hundreds of recipes. You might find the root sold fresh in the produce section of Asian markets to be used in soups and teas or used for syrups, jams, dressings, bread, cookies, cakes, and dried candy.

Ginger is normally grown in large commercial harvests since it can be used for many remedies, from adding spice to food to healing certain ailments. When you shop for ginger root, ensure that the gnarly fist-like bulb is smooth, the surface hard to the touch, and the skin not translucent.

Ginseng Tea

Ginseng is a commonly available root best known for restoration and rejuvenation. The Korean ginseng, for example, stimulates the cerebral cortex and counters exhaustion and extreme illness. It replenishes depleted energy and body fluids and is capable of removing toxins from the body. The health benefits of ginseng tea, derived from the ginseng plant root, include a boosted immune system, and a reduced risk of developing cancer. A beloved product of Korea, India, China, Japan, and America, this globally known herbal tea also has the reputation of decreasing stress. According to the American Academy of Family Physicians, this tea possesses many advantages and anti-carcinogenic properties due to the natural chemicals called ginsenosides present in the root. According to sites like sciencedaily.com and webmd.com, ginseng is also beneficial for managing diabetes.

Green Tea

Whatever benefits the heart also benefits the brain. Although tea has been linked with health benefits around the world, its medicinal properties have been investigated scientifically within the United States only in recent years. According to medical journals, green tea is reported to prevent heart-related problems, decrease cholesterol and high blood pressure, and improve the flow of blood. Green tea appears to help people with diabetes and Alzheimer's disease by blocking the formation of plaques.

where to find peace so you can live like mad

Green tea is the best food source for a group called catechins. Catechin is a type of antioxidant that lowers cholesterol and blood pressure and can protect against an unhealthy diet. Studies have found a connection between drinking green tea and a reduced risk for skin, breast, lung, colon, esophageal, and bladder cancers. Health benefits are mainly due to a high content of flavonoids — one of the largest nutrient families known to scientists, and famous for its antioxidant and anti-inflammatory health benefits.

Antioxidants protect cells from damage, aids in fending off diseases, and keep blood clotting under control. Non-synthetic supplements can be quickly absorbed by the body and offer immediate results without side effects.

Ginkgo Biloba Tea

The Ginkgo Biloba tree, native to China, is considered to be the oldest living tree on Earth. Recognized from similar fossils, studies have shown that this tree dates back to 270 million years ago. All parts of the Ginkgo Biloba tree can be used in treating different ailments. Its leaves, fruits, seeds, and even the bark can improve a person's health and wellness.

Made of whole or cut leaves, Ginko Biloba tea is claimed to have a high amount of antioxidants, which stimulates and enhances the blood circulation of the body. Proper circulation is a necessity for every person to live longer and function properly. To further protect against heart disease, it has been discovered that prolonged consumption of Ginkgo Biloba tea relieves restricted blood flows in the fingers and toes, and inhibits the formation of plaque in blood clotting thus minimizes blood coagulation, cramps, and headaches.

Ginkgo Biloba removes toxins from bad cholesterol in small arteries and promotes proper circulation, improves the mood, and reduces lethargy. People who regularly drink Ginkgo Biloba tea often report a good sense of well-being and mental alertness. This herb has also been used for overall brain functioning, including the treatment of depression, anxiety, hearing loss, concentration, memory, and hormonal imbalances. The antioxidant properties are also known to repair cells, slow down the effects of aging and reduce the risk of dementia, heart disease, stroke, cancer, and many other severe conditions.

The exponential increase in the energy level of the human body is another one of the leading benefits of Ginkgo Biloba. Apart from that, it can serve as a potential curative for sleep deprivation and even the restoration of damaged cells. Other benefits have to do with the prevention and treatment of stroke by minimizing the formation of clots in the arteries and improving blood flow to major organs, including the brain. The increased blood flow is an advantage for the brain's neurotransmitters. Moreover, diseases such as Alzheimer's and Parkinson's (associated with uncontrollable shaking, reduced coordination and balance) are treated.

Interactive Element: Herbal Tea Ritual

Activity: Prepare an herbal tea from ingredients mentioned in the chapter (e.g., ginger, ginseng). Create a ritual around drinking the tea, focusing on mindfulness and gratitude. Record your experience and any changes in mood or energy.

Example: "I made a ritual of preparing and drinking ginseng tea every evening. The process of brewing the tea and the calming effects of ginseng helped me unwind and reflect on my day with a sense of tranquility and gratitude."

TACTICAL BREATHING

One of my sister's elderly patients had been yelled at by her father over coughing spasms when she was just a child. He would scream at her to "stop coughing," and often she would run away in the cornfields to escape his angry attention. During her childhood, he also verbally abused her for other things. Most hurtful was when he accused her of coughing as if she purposely did so to bother him. On top of this father's verbal abuse, it turned out their house was infected with mold, including her bedroom. Today she has Chronic Obstructive Pulmonary Disease (COPD), a chronic inflammatory lung disease that causes obstructed airflow. Now that she is an elder, she has reactively held onto the habit of coughing and then quickly apologizing for it. Not only that, because she did not feel safe to allow her body to properly and effectively take care of itself, she often tried to suppress the urge to cough even though it is a natural way for her lungs to rid itself of phlegm or other toxins.

Everyone breathes (of course!), but some of us were never told how to breathe most efficiently. Others of us were punished for making noise. The consequence is that we might breathe fast and/or high in the chest. Shallow breathing is restrictive, it increases anxiousness, and it fuels the body's adverse stress reactions. Slow and conscious breathing is an essential strategy to stay calm to counter this. Slow, deep breathing prompts a relaxation response, calming the body, and centering the mind. It also increases the blood's oxygen level, adding to our performance potential.

Are you breathing correctly? To find out, try this: place one hand on your chest and the other on your tummy just below your ribs. Now breathe. Which hand moves? If it's the hand on your chest, your breathing is too shallow.

The goal is to see your hand move while it is rested on your abdomen. Slowly count to five while you inhale deeply. Seek to expand your abdomen instead of your chest. If you have trouble, try it lying on your back. With a little practice and persistence, you are able to automatically shift into deep conscious breathing. You can practice by placing a book on your tummy. Watch it move up and down as you inhale and exhale.

Once you learn the technique, you can breathe easy during stressful times like in the middle of a traffic jam, right before you handle the next irate customer or boss, or during an important presentation.

Many people are aware of the way breathing is taught in preparation for childbirth, but such breathing can be used for other challenges and activities. When practiced several times a day, conscious tactical breathing becomes natural. Relax neck and shoulders, breathe in through your nose, and then exhale through pursed lips as if gently blowing out a candle flame. Imagine the candle slightly flickering for four seconds. Breathe in through your nose for four counts and out through pursed lips.

During stressful situations, you can use this simple technique called pursed lips breathing to calm your nerves. Pursed-lip breathing is a conventional method taught during a therapy session. It is typically suggested for those who cope with chronic lung disease or pain management.

It is important to permit ourselves to breathe consciously and tactically, especially when we need to endure times of duress. To do so expands our lungs (and our awareness), and expels a stagnant past.

where to find peace so you can live like mad

If you are not as agile as most or if you have physical limitations (like my dad after his injury), gentle movements can also stimulate and aid our breathing. Qigong (also spelled Ch'i Kung and pronounced chee gung) is a subtle system of body movement and empowerment that are part of traditional therapy routinely practiced in Asia. Qi means a life force whose existence and properties serve as the basis of eastern philosophy, beginning more than 4000 years ago. (I like to refer to qi as the breath of life.) Gong means work or practice. The practice uses the movement of the body and the alignment of conscious breathing to maintain and restore the body and mind. Modern practitioners added meditation or what they call circulating qi based on the three primary Eastern philosophies of Confucianism, Taoism, and Buddhism, along with traditional Chinese medicine and martial arts.

Qigong is recognized to be a central basis of China's cultural heritage and one of its national treasures. Children are taught it is essential to care for the body and mind and that self-negligence causes sickness. Living balanced between sensible and sensitive, forms the answer to how to walk the walk. This subtle and gentle exercise intends to generate, store, and reinforce energy—rather than burn off energy.

Qigong is the "yang" application or skill of working with the body's life energy. It is a combination of breathing methods, meditation, and movement to cleanse, strengthen, and circulate the life energy to bring the body back into balance and promote good health. The accompanying breathwork allows us to take-in life-giving oxygen and breathe out harmful toxins, sometimes caused by a hurtful past. Meditation can free the mind of unhealthy thoughts and improve mental clarity, focus, and the ability to concentrate.

The most familiar aspect of qigong for most people will be the movements. Some people practice the art alone as a simple exercise rather than a healing path, but the results are the same: the change of the energy around the body to improve health and vitality. Elders, adults, and even children gain benefits from practicing various exercises. Both have been attributed to the quality of life regardless of age.

The art of qigong involves practicing posture, breathing, meditation, and slow, controlled exercises. Any type of movement, including gentle eastern-based exercises, in addition to prevention and treatment, completes the holistic health of the individual.

Whereas traditional martial arts is referred to as hard qigong, tai chi is considered to be soft "yin" qigong. Today it is not uncommon to find tai chi masters visiting wellness, community and senior centers in the United States. In fact, during the 1990s, a tai chi master gave a weekly class at one of the retirement facilities my sister worked at when she was just starting her job. Patients in wheelchairs circled the man as he demonstrated each position, and explained the effects on the body's circulation. Then the master moved around the room, assisting some of the elderly patients with their positioning and movements. It was shocking for my sister to be able to feel the energy moving around her hands and body.

All of us can exercise our way out of low energy. I like to catch the warmth from the sunshine and the cool breeze. I've also tried yoga and other forms of stretching to activate achy or stiff muscles. At the same time, this exercise promotes focused attention and mindfulness, a form of attention that pulls the brain into the "now," centered and calm. Dancing to my favorite songs from the 1980s leave me laughing and feeling revitalized. Walking, jogging, running, or swimming are also beneficial forms of fitness used to enhance my emotional, mental, and physical health. These are some of the best ways to raise my mood. We can often lift our mood with various types of movement.

Think about fun childhood activities that can be used today. What makes you feel good? Do you ice or roller skate? Do you enjoy riding a bike or exploring the landscape on a refreshing stroll around the neighborhood? The result is an oxygenated brain and an elevated mood. It may be one of the most effective modes of operation when it comes to

where to find peace so you can live like mad

extending the life and clearing the mind of sabotaging thoughts.

Interactive Element: Conscious Breathing

Activity: Practice tactical breathing techniques three times a day for a week, place one hand on your chest and the other on your tummy just below your ribs. Now breathe. Which hand moves? If it's the hand on your chest, your breathing is too shallow.

The goal is to see your hand move while it is rested on your abdomen. Slowly count to five while you inhale deeply. Seek to expand your abdomen instead of your chest.

If you have trouble, try it lying on your back. You can practice by placing a book on your tummy. Watch it move up and down as you inhale and exhale. Record any changes in stress levels, mental clarity, or emotional stability in a journal.

Example: "Practicing tactical breathing three times a day helped me manage my stress levels. Inhale for four counts, hold for four, exhale for four, and pause for four. This technique calmed my mind and body, especially during stressful moments, and improved my overall well-being."

VITAMINS AND MINERALS: Some herbs can be very calming and invigorating, offering an extra boost to the body's foundation. If there is any suspicion that a depleted emotional or physical state may be the result of a worn system, we might benefit from researching the best multivitamins and essential mineral supplements to nourish the body, including bones, muscles, and all bodily operations. A healthy body can uplift the mood naturally.

FOOD IS MEDICINE

A few years in a row now, my husband and two daughters planted an embarrassing surplus of seeds into two backyard plots. We used muffin tins to map out the placements before scattering kernels onto the earth and then covered and watered. We bought a variety of fruits, vegetables, and herb seeds and sprinkled them into the ground, unsure if anything would happen from this activity. I personally never had a green thumb whatsoever. In fact, my house plants typically wilted and died despite their location next to the kitchen sink!

Maybe because my expectations were so low, but I was amazed by the abundance we were able to harvest months into the future! Because of my disbelief that anything good could come from planting, I was especially delighted to see edible crops pop up! Come summer, we had so much produce we could not eat it all, thus needing to pack and give a good amount of the surplus. Some of our crops grew to unimaginable heights like the red leaf lettuce, which, because we could not pick and eat salads fast enough, had grown into five foot trees. Other produce, like the corn stalks were so abnormal, we laughed out loud when we shucked the cob ears, and found the distorted produce in its organic state. Some were long, and others were short, and the great majority had missing kernels. But they still tasted fine. Each cob would have been immediately tossed out of grocery stores due to the odd shapes and sizes. LOL. It was fun to see the stalks protected by perfectly fine looking green ears at least from the exterior.

My suggestion is to make planting a fun activity or just plain exploration. Don't expect anything. Don't make it a chore, but rather an adventure for the entire family to see if anything happens. It may seem impracticable (especially if you believe you do not have a green thumb—like me), but it is shockingly possible to reap the rewards of seeding, cultivating and yielding your own garden produce. I've inadvertently discovered that gardening can be an exciting hobby. If you don't have space outside, try a small pot indoors at first. We planted only herbs at first and surprisingly we saw sprouts quickly, within days! Later on they can be moved outdoors and can grow exponentially.

Practitioners often prescribe herbs to help relax or calm the patient. This is called tonic herbalism, and some popular ingredients are most likely already in your kitchen. It is no coincidence that organic ingredients are some of the main ingredients. Warm foods maintain health and restore stability from depleted energy.

***

Harvesting your own garden can also be therapeutic and bring forth natural healing tonic. Earthly produce as preventative medicine dates back thousands of years. Easterners have long considered food to be the source of health, wealth, and well-being. Certain fruits and vegetables aid in the balancing of various body ailments and assist with keeping the body functioning proficiently and at its optimum. Yin produce is believed to lower the body's metabolism, while the yang produce is said to increase metabolism. A balanced diet consists of grains, nuts, fruits, vegetables, and a smaller percentage of meats.

Produce is then further categorized by five types of taste: pungent, salty, bitter, sweet, and sour. Each taste has a direct effect on an organ, and when consumed in moderation, each organ benefits in one way or another, but overconsumption can cause detrimental effects to the associated organ. This is what it means when they refer to disease as an imbalance in energy.

Gifts from Mother Nature have been used to strengthen the immune system, inhibit the growth of tumors, manage blood pressure, and a multitude of other advantages. Below are a few small examples, but every fruit, vegetable, and herb contains beneficial nutrients. The plants are also packaged as teas, and some are used for soup bases. For instance, the black and red Reishi mushrooms strengthen the immune system, increase the vitality of white blood cells, and emphasize the impact of antioxidants. For stress, Reishi mushrooms alleviate insomnia and are soothing. Lotus seed tones the kidney and spleen and eases diarrhea, stimulating appetite and has a sweet to neutral taste. Licorice root is used to detoxify, cool, and invigorate the body. It is used as a pain reliever and can regulate the action of other herbs.

According to Asia's primary philosophy in the field of medicine, universal life force or energy called chi or qi pervades the entire human body. The body's unseen energy, known as meridians, flows smoothly throughout making for healthy circulation, methodically prompting the individual to be vivacious and healthy. When there are irregularities in the circulation, a setback occurs. Therefore, to remain healthy, the current of qi must be maintained.

Because all of life is interconnected, physical pain, conditions in the body, emotions, and the thinking process all influence each other. This is the reason people who experience chronic pain might also be frequently depressed.

> "The principle of yin and yang is the foundation of the entire universe. It underlies everything in creation."
>
> -The Yellow Emperor

GOING BACK TO ZEN

The Taoist symbol often seen to represent parts of Asia symbolizes how the universe functions. The paisley shapes within the circle correspond to the interaction of two energies called Yin and Yang; they cannot exist without each other, nor are they completely black or white. The curved line through the center of the circle reminds us of the constant change of balance between the two harmonizing forces, which represent the opposite principles of the universe.

Yin, the unseen element, corresponds to the feminine power and is related to the metaphysical (or spiritual): dark, passive, afterlife, small, and night. Yang, the physical component, corresponds to the masculine and related to active, light, birth, life and day.

The cyclical nature of Yin and Yang means several things in eastern philosophy; all experiences transform into their opposite in an eternal cycle of exchange. Since one principle produces the other, all of life has within itself the seed of the opposite state. For example, illness has the seeds of health, and health contains the seeds of illness. Even though an opposite may not appear to be present, nothing is entirely devoid of its contradictory state. The dot in the center of each of the yin and yang paisley symbol signifies that within the masculine, a kernel of the feminine is present and with potential and vice versa. Another way to look at it could be this: within the physical lies a spark of the metaphysical, and within the metaphysical, there lies a spark of the physical. Each side has equal value. In fact, one cannot live without the other. Or, for the advantage of holistic health, both sides must be acknowledged for balance and harmony to occur.

The goal is to nourish the body with a range of benefits, especially from eating, to maintain immune system support, and rebalance the body's qi (energy). A belief in nature shapes how the body manages itself. The body has three physical components: blood, qi, and moisture; these and other vital components are taken into consideration, along with two non-physical factors: Spirit and essence. The interaction of

where to find peace so you can live like mad

these five components is believed to have a significant impact on the body's health.

In the case of hypertension, a mixture of hawthorn, linden blossom, yarrow, and valerian might be recommended. The yarrow here is a diuretic, while the rest act as relaxing agents. Hypertension with a headache is treated with an additional wood betony, while stress involves the usage of Siberian ginseng and skullcap.

Arthritis and inflammation can also be treated with greens. Plants like Astragalus have been used to treat the common cold, fever, and influenza, among other conditions, plus stabilize the immune system. Schisandra vine has been rumored to prevent diarrhea, cough, and stress. Echinacea is also known to beat a cold or flu and is now manufactured into teas and cough drops.

These are small samples of nature's bounty. Simple remedies used in the past, as well as body care, can seed potential record-breaking significance and have vastly contributed to the maintenance of the holistic health of humanity. The history and usage of herbalism originated many thousands of years ago, but only recently became acknowledged in the west. In this form of treatment, nutrition balances and treats specific conditions depending on the cause or the type of affected area. From this ancient viewpoint, each plant carries an energetic component, and this determines which remedy can address a particular issue. The energies of the body are classified as cold, cool, warm, and hot. The prescribed herbs are typical of the opposite heat from the disrupted energy.

When the body is in symmetry, health is predominant; when Yin and Yang are imbalanced, ailment occurs. Once the Chinese medicine doctor has diagnosed the nature of an imbalance, he or she aims to restore equilibrium through a variety of natural approaches, typically using food as medicine and recommending a lifestyle change. As the balance is restored in the body and the immune cared for and strengthened, so too the mental and physical health of the individual.

Interactive Element: Healing Recipes

Activity: Try a new healing recipe and prepare it. Reflect on how the food makes you feel physically and emotionally. Share the recipe and your experience with a friend or family member.

Example: "I prepared a ginger tea with fresh ginger, honey, and lemon. Drinking it slowly, I felt a soothing warmth spread through my body. This simple recipe not only boosted my immune system but also made me feel nurtured and cared for."

NEEDLES AND KNOTS

Crazy, but it's true. A bunch of pins and needles made me smile again. One day I was afflicted with a nerve problem on one side of my face called Bell's Palsy. This means that, like a power outage, the nerves on one side of my face sedated, causing me to be unable to make facial expressions on one side due to the nerve damage. The occurrence emerged only slightly at first. When I drank from a straw or sipped from a soup spoon, a little liquid seeped through drooped lips, but I didn't think much of it. My husband, too, noticed something was off at lunch that afternoon, but merely asked if I had done something different with my hair—like did I get a haircut? (We laugh about it now.)

I had yet to look in the mirror at that point in the day, and I didn't sense the lazy side of my face. Eventually, the affected nerves on one side of my face deadened, and as a consequence, the muscles stiffened from the nerve damage like an electrical failure. I was unable to blink my eyelid on that side and didn't sense the unusual circumstances. By dinner time, the muscles on only one side of my face had completely failed, and that's when my two teenage daughters took notice. We went to a local clinic but learned that there really isn't a remedy for cases such as this.

Fortunately, my in-laws from Vietnam came to my rescue, offering an alternative solution, suggesting that I try acupuncture since it was known to resolve this crisis for others there. Looking back, I'm surprised I didn't panic or become distressed. My mind remained calm and strangely at peace.

Acupuncture is based on yin and yang philosophy. Complementary and inseparable forces within the human body represent all of nature and the universe. Total health is achieved by maintaining a balanced state through vital pathways that allow for the flow of qi. A series of twelve primary meridian streams and eight secondary streams connect over two thousand acupuncture points along the body.

As more and more Western scientists and researchers acknowledge the healing benefits of Traditional Chinese Medicine, it is finally accepted in the United States to be a proficient additional treatment. This acceptance excites those of us who find alternative and complementary medicine to be significant sources of preventative and therapeutic care for lessening pain, warding against illnesses, for overall restoration, and even recovery from mysterious flukes of nature.

I was cured by about a month's worth of treatments consisting of a one hour visit twice a week. I had no idea that over a quarter of the world's population already turned to acupuncture, acupressure, deep massage, Qigong, and herbal medicine for medical treatments. The idea is to tap into the body's qi and keep it flowing to avoid illness. Any blockages can manifest in the body being out of sync with itself.

Acupuncture originated in China thousands of years ago and is one of many methods around the world now used as a valuable medical procedure. The treatment is known for not only relieving immediate pain, but reputed to be a preventative agent against imbalances because it realigns the body's energy system.

The treatment, one of the oldest medical systems in human history, belongs to a community of procedures to stimulate the body's anatomy through balancing the energy flow via invisible meridian channels from specific acupuncture locations. The placement of needles releases a range of the body's hormones, like antibodies, stimulating the immune system, endorphins, feel-good chemicals in the brain and improving blood flow to help it heal.

Investigations are popping up all over the world providing evidence on its usefulness in many areas of healthcare. Studies reveal that it serves to complement standard care and provide pain relief, and improves mobility of joints caused by arthritis inflammation. One theory proposes that acupuncture produces its effects through regulating the nervous system, inducing the release of endorphins and immune system cells at specific sites on the body. There is also the theory that acupuncture alters the brain chemistry by changing the neurotransmitters.

The treatment was founded on the belief that to remain healthy, our vital energy flow must maintain its balance. The necessary flow could be out of sync, but we can still appear healthy. It is in this capacity that acupuncture serves as preventive medicine. Checking and balancing the flow of energy on the body's meridian points is comparable to maintaining your car before anything happens.

What to Expect During an Acupuncture Treatment

Acupuncture is one of several popular alternative therapies in which all disorders can be traced to a Chi imbalance. The treatment is regarded to be one of the most common and oldest worldwide. Pinpointing (no pun intended), the body's blocked centers release the bound qi and allows it to flow naturally; it is then that the body can restore and heal itself.[1]

On the first diagnosis, acupuncturists usually ask new clients to fill out a personal health record. The client might answer questions on health issues, age, diet, emotional and

---

1. Those considering acupuncture might want to initially consult a doctor or healthcare professional for advice on their conditions and then make a decision on a treatment plan that makes the most sense for the individual. Organizations such as the American Academy of Medical Acupuncturists offer a list of qualified and certified acupuncturists and practitioners.

psychological profile, sleeping patterns, and overall lifestyle and regular activities during the initial interviews. The individual should also inform the practitioner of any current medications and treatments. The more information the acupuncturist has, the better one can determine where the qi is blocked.

You might see the practitioner evaluate pulse points or even glance at the tongue to establish the health of the individual or the status of the twelve meridians. A diagnosis is then given before treatment commences.

During treatments, the acupuncturist gently inserts thin pliable and disposable needles just beneath the surface of the skin along the invisible meridian lines indicative of a specific channel that has to do with the ailment. Each point corresponds to a particular organ system that links with yin or yang energy, and each point is controlled manually or by electrical stimulation.

While the practitioner makes the diagnosed insertions into one or more connected pathways, the patient typically rests on a massage table facing the ceiling. The needles are inserted while the patient remains in a quiet and private room for about an hour. You may also have someone with you while you receive the treatment. Other influences attributed to the therapy include the release of endorphins, connections of neurotransmitters, and the promotion of circulation. The interest in acupuncture increased after the numerous side effects of conventional medicine became apparent. The modality addresses many common ailments and undesirable conditions and has been utilized to treat the following health issues without side effects:

•Addictions •Allergies •Anxiety •Arthritis •Asthma •Bell's Palsy •Carpal Tunnel Syndrome •Chemotherapy side effects •Chronic Pain •Colds •Depression •Headache •Low-Back Pain •Infertility •Menstrual Cramps •Migraines •Muscular Problems •Postoperative nausea •Sinusitis •Tennis Elbow

I still have some silly photos of me with half a smiling face, but I have recovered from the nerve damage completely. Every once in a while, I might feel my face twitch, but when that occurs, I'll make myself a small cup of magnesium tea, and it seems to take care of the problem. I do the same if I experience a tight leg cramp, which used to occur after I would go for walks.2

Interactive Element: Acupressure Practice

Activity: Learn about basic acupressure points and practice a simple routine to relieve stress or minor aches. Document your experience and any changes you feel in a journal.

Example: "I learned basic acupressure points for stress relief and practiced them daily. Pressing the point between my thumb and index finger for a few minutes reduced my anxiety significantly and brought a sense of calm and balance."

---

2. If you are squeamish about needles, acupressure is an alternative modality mentioned in the next chapter. I waited until I absolutely needed an acupuncture treatment before I decided to go ahead. I was at the point where it appeared to be the only option. I'm not saying that this modality would help everyone, but I was pleased with my own healing result.

HANDS-ON HEALING

Like acupuncture, acupressure focuses on moving chi through energy points called meridians to help the entire body function, restore itself, and remain stress-free. This hands-on healing method is perfect for those who do not like needles, and for anyone who wishes to heal themselves through another method of energy therapy. Acupressure is a noninvasive method that has been claimed to reduce stress levels, general aches and suffering, and aid in recovery from injury and surgery. It has also been safe for children and used to reduce nausea and vomiting.

Acupressure consists of gentle pressure from hands, thumbs, or forefingers. The concept of chi is central in Eastern philosophy. As mentioned in previous chapters, when the chi is blocked, it can result in a build-up of pressure that can further grow into an imbalance or un-ease, (some say if unaddressed can devolve into dis-ease). We all know the pain of inner turmoil!

Acupuncture and acupressure share the network of vital energy points situated along meridian channels throughout the body. Pain and problems in one part of the body are controlled and alleviated by meridians in other parts of the body. Whereas acupuncture uses thin needles, acupressure uses hand placements to manipulate the energies, release pressure, and open blocked channels, allowing for the qi to flow freely once more, leading to pain relief, better body function, and a release of toxins.

GOING BACK TO ZEN

Practitioners are trained to determine which energetic pools and channels are associated with locations to free pain or illness. They then apply gentle-to-firm pressure to alleviate pain and reduce various symptoms from the following:

•*Allergies* •*Anxiety Attacks* •*Asthma* •*Nervousness* •*Tension* •*Migraine Headaches* •*Jaw Pain* •*Toothaches Earache* •*Backache* •*Joint pain* •*Colds and Flu* •*Sore Throat* •*Sinus Infection* •*Depression* •*Insomnia* •*Fainting* •*Hiccups* •*Improve* •*Memory and Concentration* •*Angina* •*Heart Palpitations* •*High Blood Pressure* •*Elimination* •*Heartburn* •*Stomach Ache* •*Cramps* •*Hot Flashes* •*Pregnancy Discomfort* •*Incontinence* •*Urinary retention* •*Nose bleeding*

My absolute preferred look at hands-on-healing comes from the founder of the Jin Shin Do (JSD) Foundation for Bodymind Acupressure, and author of one of my favorite books, The Joy of Feeling: BodyMind AcupressureTM. Iona Marsaa Teeguarden uses various gentle hand placements as a tool for recovery along the body's biological meridian lines in conjunction with psychology and talk therapy to release pent up energetic imbalances. The qi carries information much like the color spectrum and radio waves, and are electromagnetic in nature, an important human aspect. Each organ is associated with energy in motion, and if there is an imbalance, then certain symptoms will occur. When these emotions become excessive or turned inward or outward, they can develop into chronic and cause disease. At first, we might merely feel uneasy, but if we do not release the emotion, it can affect our physicality. We need to acknowledge unhealthy and invasive environments. If we seek to maintain health and overcome potential illnesses, the imbalances can be corrected. This is why allowing for ourselves and others to be angry (or any other mood) is necessary for the effort for healing. Anger, like any heavy emotion, needs to be released in a healthy and hearty manner instead of being repressed and stagnant, ultimately blocking the flow of healthy qi. The grief, fear, sadness, worry, anger, etc. that do not have

where to find peace so you can live like mad

opportunities for expression prevent the body from being free of pain and sorrow. Eventually, the energy builds up, and we carry the burdens and the toll wherever we go (sometimes for decades).

According to ancient and traditional Chinese philosophy and medicine, these organs hold the following emotions, resulting in the following imbalances.

Interactive Element: Self-Massage Techniques

Activity: Follow a tutorial on self-massage techniques for stress relief. Practice these techniques daily for a week and note any improvements in your physical or emotional well-being.

Example: "Using a tutorial, I practiced self-massage on my neck and shoulders. The gentle pressure and movements released tension and improved my mood. This daily practice became a cherished moment of self-care and relaxation."

HEART
Houses: Shen or Soul
Emotion: joy
Imbalanced: mania and despair

SPLEEN
Houses: Yi or thinking
Emotion: worry
Imbalanced: dwelling, mulling

LUNG
Houses: Po or reaction
Emotion: sadness
Imbalanced: grief, detachment

KIDNEYS
Houses: Zhi or memory
Emotion: fear
Imbalanced: insecure self-doubt and panic

LIVER
Houses: Hun or self-control
Emotion: anger
Imbalanced: resentment, rage

HOLDERS OF LIFE KNOWLEDGE

Before I began to study international adoption and write about my experiences, I fell in love with eastern philosophy and world religions. This love pulled me through when my research led me to tough findings and rough patches, particularly when uncovering the corruption found in so many areas. The wisdom and philosophy derived from the past might pull you through. The wealth of natural wonder I have gathered from the east inspires me to share this interest with you.

In Ayurvedic medicine, the primary energy centers of the body are said to consist of seven chakras (also called vortexes). Chakra is the Sanskrit word for four-wheel. They are located at the base of the spine to the top of the head. Each chakra is equally crucial for the body's optimal functioning according to the Ayurvedic healing tradition.

The human body has seven primary chakras that correspond with emotional and spiritual aspects, according to practitioners of this particular energetic healing. Each vortex relates to a region of the body, similar to the way traditional Chinese medicine addresses specific ailments, colors, and elements with emotions connected to each organ. The chakras hold vibrational frequencies and represent symbols. Each energy center must be vibrating at the proper frequency independent of one another for the entire body to vibrate in harmony.

GOING BACK TO ZEN

The chakras are imagined as spinning from front to back and running along the spine in the center of the body. The seven primary chakras balance the human energy system, and each is associated with a color, and a particular energy field, starting from the base of the spine and working to the top of the head. The chakras are:

The Crown Chakra (white)
The Third Eye Chakra (violet)
The Throat Chakra (Indigo)
The Heart Chakra (green)
The Solar Plexus Chakra (yellow)
The Sacral Chakra (orange)
The Root Chakra (red)

The colors are associated with the rainbow starting with red at the base of the spine to purple at the crown of the head. Chakras become blocked from a lack of nurturing and protection caused by losses, conflict, accidents, injuries, and heavy emotions like anger, worry, fear, and grief, which arrive from unexpected and traumatic events.

The Root (1st) Chakra, associated with the color red, is located at the base of the spine near the tailbone. The energy has to do with foundation, safety, security, stability, protection, and basic survival needs, such as food, water, and shelter. This chakra governs the spinal column, kidneys, legs, feet, rectum, and immune system. This deals with the first family, tribal connection with ancestral roots, and the relationship with the earth. Someone with a healthy root chakra tends to be very secure, stable, and grounded. When this chakra is out of balance, it may lead to lower back pain, varicose veins, leg cramps, rectal conditions, as well as immune-related disorders. Emotional imbalances may include lower self-esteem, insecurity, or family concerns.

The Sacral (2nd) Chakra—associated with the color orange, is located two inches below the navel. The vortex relates to sexuality, sociability, relationships, passion for life, friends, love, possessions, power, and joy. The energy also has to do with procreation (or creation) and reproduction (or production). Someone with a dominant orange aura is usually a risk taker and outgoing.

The Solar Plexus (3rd) Chakra, associated with the color yellow, is located in the middle of the body where the ribs separate. The energy field surrounding this chakra has to do with openness to self-esteem, to gut-level intuition, and being physically in harmony with mind and body. The energies between lower and upper areas have to do with the body's functions, and also the environment. With a healthy yellow chakra, you are in tune with your willpower, emotions, and gut responses. People with dominant yellow auras tend to be active and love the outdoors.

The Heart (4th) Chakra, associated with the color green, is located at the heart. The energy has to do with empathy, love, and compassion. A balanced chakra is harmonious and receptive to all of life—even those who disagree and disagreeable circumstances. It is also better able to discern between shallow and superficial appearances versus honesty, kindness, and genuine truth. A healthy heart aligns the spirit with mind and body and adapts to finding common ground in diverse situations. The healthy individual generously gives and receives a clean dose of attentiveness and affection to oneself and others.

The Throat (5th) Chakra, associated with the color blue, is associated with the throat. A balanced chakra speaks fearlessly and honestly truth to power. When centered, communication and creativity connect with the greater self and community. A balanced chakra allows for the individual to speak honestly and with sincerity.

The Third Eye (6th) Chakra, associated with the color indigo, is located between and slightly above the eyebrows. The energy has to do with insightfulness: being able to see beneath the surface of things and also the bigger picture. A healthy chakra allows for an understanding of individuals and groups with greater clarity and empathy to look behind misconstrued messages and false witnesses. Openness to knowledge, the trust of your intuition, and inner guidance are benefits of a healthy third eye.

The Crown (7th) Chakra, associated with the color purple, is located at the top of the head. The energy has to do with being open to spiritual or universal oneness. When receptive, meditation can allow for us to resonate and unite with the authentic self (and "all that is") in connection with the universal plane of existence. A healthy chakra allows for the individual to know that all are significant members of the natural realm of sacred energy life force. In the end, we all matter.

To balance chakras and harness energy, therapists funnel sacred life force energy through their hands. Massage, crystals, gemstones, chanting, visualization, imagination, meditation, and movement are common tools used to cleanse away toxic energies.

Sometimes dormant subtle energy is referred to as Kundalini, a Sanskrit word meaning "circular." Imagine a coiled snake or a spring at the base of the spine. The vital force has the potential to stay compressed or rise to the surface. Prescribed meditations and exercises can rouse this primal force up the spine to the seventh chakra. At its fully informed and awakened state, the personality of the practitioner is transformed. A "thousand-petal lotus" depicts enlightenment at the crown of the head. Insightfulness offers information from the inside out and provides a brighter point of view aligned with the universal oneness.

The early healing philosophy forming the basis of Ayurvedic medicine is a collection of Sanskrit scriptures known as Vedas. While Ayur means "life" or "vital power," Veda means "knowledge" or "wisdom." The art of chakra healing has been used for centuries to revitalize the body's vital centers. An energized body and a happier, more peaceful individual results. (Ayurveda remained the predominant form of care in India until the British colonial government tried to suppress it during the nineteenth century.)

> "IMAGINATION IS MORE IMPORTANT THAN KNOWLEDGE. FOR KNOWLEDGE IS LIMITED TO ALL WE NOW KNOW AND UNDERSTAND, WHILE IMAGINATION EMBRACES THE ENTIRE WORLD, AND ALL THERE EVER WILL BE TO KNOW AND UNDERSTAND."
>
> --ALBERT EINSTEIN

Meditating on each chakra may also be used to open vitality centers and improve the body's flow of positive energy. During meditation, visualize each of the chakras starting with the base and working the way up to the crown chakra located at the top of the head. By imagining the movement of energy from center to center, we assist with the removal of blockages that could be causing pain or suffering and sabotaging the individual from starting or attaining goals.

Many believe that the chakras have the power to transform and brighten life. Because the chakras govern every organ and system in the body, chakra healing has numerous health benefits influencing the heart, lung, brain, immune, and digestive function, and may also relieve depression, anxiety, and other mood imbalances. When our chakras are in sync, we become attuned to higher levels of consciousness.

Numerous natural remedies affect the vibration of each spinning wheel, and that's where chakra balancing comes into play. Gemstones, the human voice, music, chants, mantras, and meditation bring the frequency of the chakras back into proper vibrational alignment. For example, the root chakra is affected by red gemstones, like hematite, onyx, ruby, and garnet. During a chakra healing, the practitioner may use one or all of these chakra stones to cleanse the root chakra and bring it into harmony akin to brightening up the space. In today's world, this has been translated into color therapy or even light therapy. Meditate on colors, or on light, and see what happens to your mood!

Interactive Element: Chakra Visualization and Balancing

Activity: Chakra Balancing Meditation
Step 1: Find a quiet place where you won't be disturbed. Sit comfortably with your spine straight and close your eyes.

Step 2: Take a few deep breaths, inhaling peace and exhaling stress.

Step 3: Visualize each of the seven chakras in your body, starting from the root chakra at the base of your spine and moving upwards to the crown chakra at the top of your head.

Step 4: Spend a few moments focusing on each chakra, imagining it glowing brightly in its respective color: red for root, orange for sacral, yellow for solar plexus, green for heart, blue for throat, indigo for third eye, and violet for crown.

Step 5: As you focus on each chakra, visualize any blockages or negative energy being released and the chakra spinning freely and brightly.

Step 6: *After balancing all the chakras, imagine a stream of white light flowing from your crown chakra down through all the chakras, cleansing and harmonizing them.*

Example: *"Today, I practiced the chakra balancing meditation. I started by visualizing my root chakra glowing a vibrant red. I felt a sense of grounding and stability. Moving up to my sacral chakra, I saw it glowing orange and felt creativity and passion flow through me. At my solar plexus chakra, I visualized a bright yellow light and felt empowered and confident. My heart chakra glowed green, filling me with love and compassion. My throat chakra turned blue, helping me feel more expressive and truthful. My third eye chakra shone indigo, enhancing my intuition and insight. Finally, my crown chakra glowed violet, connecting me to a higher state of consciousness. The white light flowing through all my chakras at the end left me feeling balanced, rejuvenated, and at peace."*

MASSAGE FOR THE SOUL

Reiki, a healing art discovered by a Japanese minister, also works with energy, derived from the same pool of complementary and traditional Chinese medicine. In Japan, Rei denotes a spiritual essence that permeates all of nature and of a higher intelligence. (From the original biblical Hebrew texts, the definition of the word is "my shepherd; my companion.") The name itself suggests that the guidance of a divine source is used for healing. The Ki stands for life force energy. Like other methods of eastern medicine, Reiki symbolizes life force, which is energetically and spiritually guided. Reiki Masters use their hands as a therapeutic tool to guide the flow of energy, but they do not touch the body while influencing the chakra and meridian system. This form of hands-on healing is intended to release the flow of toxic forces and push away various bodily maladies. The principles of Reiki have been used for thousands of years, but were developed into a system in the late 19th century by Dr. Mikao Usui, also rumored to be a minister and the head of a Christian school located in Japan.

Dr. Usui's students wanted to know how Jesus healed, which prompted his research into hands-on healing. Soon, the minister became fixated on discovering how Jesus had cured the ill and infirm. He spent years studying in Christian schools, Buddhist monasteries, and temples, but he could not find an answer to the pervasive question. Eventually, he embarked on a fast that lasted for twenty-one days. At its end, Dr. Usui where to find peace so you can live like mad claimed to have received insight, which initiated his ministry of Reiki healing. He then incorporated meditation techniques, beliefs, and also symbols into his practice.

> *JUST FOR TODAY DO NOT WORRY. JUST FOR TODAY LET GO OF ANGER. CONSIDERATION FOR PARENTS, TEACHERS, AND ELDERLY. EARN YOUR LIVING HONESTLY. BE KIND TO ALL LIVING THINGS.*

Eventually, he shared his findings with Dr. Chujiro Hyashi, who, in turn, shared the data with Mrs. Hawayo Takata.

It was Mrs. Takata who brought the practice to the United States after World War II. She trained twenty-two Reiki Masters, who then shared the knowledge with thousands of others. According to Reiki philosophy, the client receives a tune-up, which leaves the person feeling at peace and with more confidence to manage life. The ki is then realigned and balanced, and the harmony restored in the client's body.

Reiki meditation typically concentrates on self-healing, the five spiritual principles, and accreditation of the healer is accomplished through a process of attunement. The primary purpose is to be able to restore and rejuvenate the universal and spiritual flow of chi. The sub-purpose is to gain emotional and physical stamina. Most of the Reiki practitioners believe that the therapy connects life force with the body. Hands are placed over traditional positions to channel sacred energy through the body for self-healing. Reiki masters are the bridge.

Reiki can also be practiced in group sessions and distance healing. In group sessions, two or more Reiki practitioners place hands over the body of another. In distance sessions, the practitioners visualize the client through the Reiki symbol. This activity can be comparable to the power of prayer.

The Reiki Master normally conducts a service in which the students imagine a symbol and hands clasped.

The Three Levels of Attunement:

Reiki I:
The Reiki Master shares the channel of energy for self-healing to open a lineage of sorts. The student is now open to receive and learn. At this time the student healers are taught the basic hand positions and the sacred symbols. The student can direct energy for others.

Reiki II:
The Reiki Master gives a second attunement to connect the student directly with the source chi, similar to a baptism. Also, student healers can teach the meaning of symbols and hand positions to practice distance or absentee healing.

Reiki III:
Most people do not consider level three Reiki until after at least six months of contemplation. Level three can take months or even years of service. The third attunement creates a permanent open channel of energy from the master to the student recipient and can be especially beneficial when paired with massage. Student healers commit to the universal power as a sacred life force. Practitioners refer to them as Reiki Masters.

Reiki is not a type of religion, but healers do establish five primary principles and work only for the greater good:

My sister's experience with Reiki

In 1997, my sister inadvertently became aware of a gentle relaxation modality and attuned to the energy from Reiki practitioners before her. The energy must have been resting dormant for the next ten years while she worked with elders at her "real" job in assisted-living facilities. But every time she picked up and read from a particular Reiki book, her hands warmed and even tingled. Reiki energy soon followed.

In 2008, my sister eventually studied on her own, and then followed up with a fellow Reiki Master under the direct lineage of Dr. Mikao Usui. Since then, driving to work or merely being around certain individuals, the heat sometimes emanates from her hands. In some cases, the flow would move upwards along the sleeve of her lower and upper arms when she provided therapy for various patients. If they requested a Reiki treatment, they would often comment during a session, "is that heat coming from you?" Many expressed how their pain subsided after she placed her hands over particular areas like their joints, wounds, or shoulders. My sister calls the treatment a "massage for the soul." Whenever she feels her hands heat up, she follows the heat to wherever it takes her.

My sister had the opportunity to give Reiki treatments to Dr. Ruth Kelly, one of Oprah Winfrey's mentors and Maya Angelou's best friend. After the session with my sister, we are permitted to report that Dr. Ruth Kelly's blood-pressure improved, among other benefits. They also became friends. The elder woman gave my sister encouraging words via text and messages, and gifted her (and me) with time and wisdom. Dr. Ruth then introduced us to her other best friend, Dr. Maxine Mimms. I was fortunate to be mentored and encouraged by the wise Dr. Mimms on the re-release of Americanized '72 (my first book). Shockingly, the elder woman complimented me on the writing of that book. As an educator, she spent her professional career advocating for less recognized, but self-motivated and action-oriented individuals, promoting dialogues and discussions which would be uncomfortable for many. She even started Evergreen College from her kitchen table! After I had published The Search for Mother Missing, I had hidden it away for almost twenty years, but Dr. Mimms saw its potential and encouraged me to make it available to the public. She understood the inner urging I had to advocate for roots, steeped deep within the core of each human being—something no human-made and fallible system should have the right to remove from any individual. I am forever grateful for the time I had with her.

Interactive Element: Guided Reiki

Activity: Participate in a guided Reiki session focused on healing and relaxation. Journal your thoughts and feelings after the session, noting any new insights or areas of peace.

Example: "I participated in a guided meditation session focused on healing. The visualization of a peaceful beach and the soothing voice of the guide brought me to a state of deep relaxation and inner peace. It was a rejuvenating experience."

ON CONNECTION & COMMUNITY

Humanity needs to rediscover the oneness that connects all of us and affirm that we are all more alike than different. We can also place value on our diversity instead of permitting disagreements to divide us.

We can band together to acknowledge, listen, and give consideration to every perspective.

A GENTLE, YET POWERFUL HEALER

Reiki energy is delicate, yet can be an effective soothing tool. My sister tells me that everyone has a different experience when it comes to relief. She has seen the most noticeable soothing outcome on joint or arthritis pain and recovery after injury and surgery—areas of pain where hot or cold packs are used. Some recipients are able to sense the heat emitting from the Reiki Master's palms. Many recipients report feeling the heat emanating from my sister's hands, and some even prefer her hands over an E-Stim (Electrical Stimulation) Machine or diathermy.

Though it is not a religion, this palm healing works with the sacred energy life force and is interpreted to be spiritual because of its alignment with nature, and attunement with the universal oneness, called by some to be divine. Some of us like to refer to this energy as God, The Way of Nature or a Universal Life Force (whatever you want to call energy in its purest form) is acknowledged and recognized as the unmanifested source. Though there are definite theories involved, the actual methods might be compared to the laying of hands practiced by healers of various religious denominations.

This modality promotes life force and relaxes, moves, and releases trapped energy, ultimately improving the health of mind, body, and spirit.

The client cannot be harmed in any way, and there are no side effects. Recipients can place boundaries, if need be, and prevent the energy from affecting themselves. For example, emotional states like rejection, trepidation, distrust, and fears will block universal energy. Reiki can be used in conjunction with Western medicine or homeopathy; the therapy does not require patients to change religions, beliefs, or points of view. The treatment is only intended to restore the body's health and well-being.

As the recipient becomes more comfortable with the practice, she may wish to share Reiki energy with friends, family members, or even pets. When doing so, it is important to try not to expect too much. What we think is right for us might be wrong for others. I like to think of myself as merely supporting someone with energy that flows through, rather than exchanging energy. The recipient can set boundaries and refuse to allow the energy to influence them. They can also block the chi (also called ki) using an unconscious disdain for the practice or the practitioner, and even (unknowingly) disliking certain parts of the culture from which the recipient might think the practitioner is from. Even though the client's cynicism and distrust is a normal part of being human, sometimes a discriminating attitude against something—whatever that may be—even unconsciously, will prevent the best possible benefits.

The responsibility of the Reiki Practitioner is only to serve as a vessel for which universal energy can flow through. The recipient is in control of whether or not they will accept or reject the flow. Reiki Masters should be able to Reiki share without draining or depleting themselves. In fact, my sister found that by giving a treatment, she can also become energized.

Just as with all energy work, Reiki is a therapeutic journey and not a destination. Take the time to sense your energy and see if there is a difference in terms of strength levels, ability to recover, and overall feeling of calm and comfort. When my sister and I first learned about energy, we would imagine ourselves playing with balls of light. At first we merely tossed them back and forth to each other for fun. Even when closing eyes, sometimes we could actually sense when that ball of energy was directed at us.

If you are looking for a Reiki Master, trust your instincts—the part of yourself that is more open, aware, and more receptive. Trust that you will be led to the right person at the right time, and stay open to the possibilities—whatever they may be. This good-natured attitude is the key to an exchange of energetic empowerment. You and the universe decide whether or not this exercise should come to fruition.

When you feel down or out, or if your energy is depleted, it might be time to consider Reiki or other forms of energy sessions like Jin Shin Do. Many people today enjoy the relaxation of the therapy like a massage for the soul, and due to its growing acceptance and success stories, word of mouth recommendations are growing. If you decide that energy therapy is the right choice for you, or if you are simply curious, it might be time to receive a treatment.

Reiki has been used all over the world to address illnesses, or recover after a surgery, and it has been reported to soothe the body, increase the body's ability to heal itself and augment calm. Studies have shown that using Reiki regularly can boost the immune system and help people bounce back from stressful situations. It has been associated with providing relief from depression, anxiety, and other frequent mood disturbances.

It is helpful to believe in the possibilities—whatever the universe decides might be completely different than our plans and expectations. I get excited learning about different healing modalities, but also accepting reality as it is so that I can work from a practical place of solidarity and peace.

My sister reminds me that healing does not necessarily occur only physically. Cures can also include a greater understanding due to insight into the situation, spiritual expansion, wisdom gained, emotional empowerment, relaxation, and peace. This type of healing had been a lesson learned during our childhoods.

Earth Energy

Another unique and beneficial visualization can be using the imagination of giving and receiving Reiki energy through the feet chakras. We have chakras on the soles of our feet that allow a life force exchange with the earth, a vital source of energy. Not only can your body benefit from the earth's natural energy system, but it is possible to receive an exchange of power that can aid in restoration.

We can understand the relationship between the vital reciprocal back and forth exchange between the earth, our energy system, and the universal life force energy by taking a glimpse at the life of a tree. Through its branches and leaves, trees reach the sun, their source of power, and they also draw in strength called universal life force energy through roots reaching deep and wide into the ground, pulling nutrients from the soil and water to ensure continued healthy growth.

This natural energy exchange is a balanced process for growth and expansion, a method that many spiritualists and naturalists have emulated in their meditation and reiki practices. We can balance earth energy and the universal life force energy to enable us to grow and evolve. As long as we have our feet firmly planted in the earth, it is okay to have our heads in the clouds.

Humans are energy centers similar to that of trees. Our body's system has many channels and centers running through it, resembling nature's network. The earth's centers of life force are linked to universal energy often found in sacred sites or unique places marked by stone circles, old trees, religious buildings, shrines, or statues. Sometimes these landmarks' energy systems are influenced by seasonal changes or newly built buildings or roads

When the ground is covered by concrete or not visible, it might be no surprise to find ourselves in a low mood, or caught in verbal exchanges and even unhealthy relationships, prompting a continual feeling of separation from heaven and earth.

GOING BACK TO ZEN

When we give or receive a Reiki treatment, our hearts and minds open through the chakra portal, drawing us towards the centers belonging deep and wide into the earth and above the heavens and beyond.[3]

Interactive Element: Self-Reiki Session

Activity: Self-Reiki Healing

Step 1: Find a quiet, comfortable place to sit or lie down where you won't be disturbed. Close your eyes and take a few deep breaths, allowing yourself to relax.

Step 2: Set an intention for your Reiki session, such as healing, relaxation, or balancing your energy.

Step 3: Begin by placing your hands gently on the top of your head. Imagine warm, healing energy flowing from your hands into your body.

Step 4: Slowly move your hands to different positions on your body, spending a few minutes at each spot. Focus on your third eye (forehead), throat, heart, solar plexus (upper abdomen), sacral (lower abdomen), and root (base of spine) chakras.

Step 5: As you hold your hands in each position, visualize the energy flowing into your body, clearing blockages and restoring balance. Feel the warmth and healing power of the energy.

---

3. My sister's website has more information on this unique modality: https://reiki.vancetwins.com/

Step 6: *Finish by placing your hands on your heart, thanking yourself for taking this time to heal and care for your well-being. Take a few deep breaths and slowly open your eyes when you are ready.*

Example: *"I dedicated 20 minutes to a self-Reiki session today. I set my intention for healing and began by placing my hands on the top of my head, feeling a gentle warmth spread through my scalp. Moving to my third eye, I visualized a clear, calming light. At my throat, I felt the energy opening up my ability to communicate clearly. My heart chakra filled with a soothing green light, bringing a sense of love and compassion. The solar plexus chakra glowed with empowering yellow energy, and the sacral chakra with creative orange light. Finally, at the root chakra, I felt a deep sense of grounding and stability. Ending with my hands on my heart, I felt a profound sense of peace and gratitude for the healing energy. This session left me feeling balanced, rejuvenated, and deeply connected to myself."*

LOST AND FOUND IN THOUGHT

To make sure I am in my best state of mind, I need to ensure that I am getting enough sleep. Sleep deprivation has been linked to numerous medical problems. It can also lead to feelings of hopelessness, other low energy moods, and can make doing routine tasks difficult. Many accidents have been caused by sleeplessness. The consequences of sleep deprivation are serious and, at times, even fatal. It is understandable to reach for pharmaceuticals in an attempt to get a satisfying rest, but these can be potentially addictive. We might assume we are depressed when our minds are just clogged up and foggy from not getting enough sleep. In the very beginning stages of writing, I would confuse just simply being tired with being depressed. If I am tired and trying to recover from the previous day, it does not matter how much time I spend writing, the quality suffers. So a priority of mine is to ensure I get quality sleep, and if not, then at least find a moment to meditate if need be. I find the best time to do my research and writing is early mornings after at least a few hours of rest when my mind is at its optimum. Everyone has their own best time.

If you are having trouble focusing on writing, meditation can serve as a safe alternative and effective sleep aid without harmful side effects. If you cannot get the sleep you need, try meditation to clear your mind. Focus on the silence, a place away from the worries of the future, and painful past experiences. If anxiety or panic attacks make you sleepless, no-thought stabilizes mood, and relieves the mind. The benefits have to do with the biochemical processes that occur in the body, like the release of endorphins, which generate a feeling of well-being. The meditation practice also increases the production of melatonin, a hormone responsible for restful sleep.

The practice of meditation benefits those who have a hard time resting. I've found that I have a difficult time falling asleep if certain issues plague my mind. Reflective writing prior to sleeping, or when I can't sleep, can help to deconstruct and release unresolved tensions that can grow into more significant problems. The practice of focused attention inward can convert poor-quality sleep into a deeper, more refreshing sleep. Many meditators say that they wake feeling more energized after spending moments focused on oneself. Additionally, meditating allows me to spend a longer time in the REM stage. This stage of sleep is crucial to the mental capacity of the brain. When we are REM sleep-deprived, we retain less information.

Meditation can also help those who suffer from Chronic Fatigue Syndrome (CFS). Several studies show that CFS patients have a deficiency of slow-wave sleep. By engaging in deep meditation, we heighten Theta and Delta brain activity. This activity is said to compensate for not enough time in the Delta (deepest) sleeping state. Because of the inner tranquility and improved creativity that meditation provides, the frequency of vivid dreams increases, especially through lucid dreaming. Meditating before bed calms nerves and aids in overcoming certain types of insomnia. Sometimes when I find myself tossing and turning in bed at night, all I need to do is listen to (by headphones) the drone of someone's voice on audio.

Or, I get up and write! Sleeplessness usually means I have something I need to say, and I need to release it. Utilize the silence. Expression through a pen or pencil works best for me. I might use conscious breathing for a few moments before I brainstorm on ideas, usually starting with whatever is plaguing my mind at the moment. At the same time, I like to listen to soft music or nature sounds to create a more serene atmosphere. If I do not feel like writing, I write a to-do list or work on an unfinished project.

***

One of my favorite places to look for solutions happens to be my own mind! The power of instinct and intuition is truly awesome and brings me joy. By going within, I am able to maximize my innate, authentic power and manifest goals into reality. Life tends to move me towards the physical equivalent of my predominant thoughts and feelings.

Sometimes it seems that thoughts are random, every so often erratic, and beyond my control. In my case, due to childhood experiences of being excluded and scolded, all too often, the programming becomes a collection of memories that create hurtful emotions and sabotaging thoughts that cause me to remain stagnant from progression. If not careful, dominant thoughts and feelings are typically negative due to dogmatic training. Unacknowledged emotions truly can take control much of the time, and it is easy to react to situations and make assumptions as the subconscious programs take over.

Real power is the conscious ability to transform automatic thinking that can dominate the mind. By assessing my thoughts, I ensure to come from a place of honesty, aligned with my soul, and therefore creating genuine life experiences based on my authentic self. The moral compass is inside. Meditation pushes my ego out of the way so that I can hear my soul's suggestions. One of the best tools to use is to question my ego using what I call reflective writing.

Reflective writing and meditation utilize my relaxed state of mind and condition my brain to respond differently to outside stimuli—situations that have caused previous reactions. When I lose myself in thought, I give myself a chance to center myself upon carefully chosen suggestions. This can be a list of simple affirmations that I mentally repeat. I might use guided meditation audios to assist me with deciding which task needs where to find peace so you can live like mad to be started next or motivate me to accomplish one of my goals.

EXAMINATION OF PROGRAMMED THOUGHTS:

This usually requires us to discern between truth and lies passed down to us as children so that we can reprogram some of that old training founded upon misconstrued beliefs to a more objective perspective and perception of ourselves, and others. A great way to determine how much we have healed is to meditate, reflect, and deconstruct past messages through journal writing.

Setting my intention for each step of the way aides me for better focus. I consciously decide what exactly I want to accomplish and then write it down. Next, I ask questions and listen for easy answers. I might spend a moment imagining myself being protected by white light from the top of my head down throughout the center of my torso and down into the ground at my feet as if washing away discouraging thoughts as the light filters through. Then I write answers to the questions previously asked. If the thoughts are considerate and loving for all of humanity, I assume I am on the right track. This is how intuition speaks to me. I particularly watch out for my ego. I try to trust that I will be given solutions that are right for me. And if there is only silence, no worries, I accept that the answers will arrive when they are ready or when I'm ready. For the time being, maybe silence is all that is needed. I interpret this silence as moments of peace, and maybe this is all that is needed for me to manage the day. Sometimes words can get in the way of feeling bliss and comfort.

One of the main things I try to keep in mind is not to verbally beat myself up for being different. Each human has their own individualistic and exclusive traits — similar to a thumbprint —and no one is better than the other. The problem (battle and even war) comes knocking when we (or others) do not value our unique take on life. From being lost in thought (even while meditating), I've found value in my distinctive strengths. All humans use different methods to accomplish tasks, and not one is better than another. This current diversity makes for a great multidimensional environment and has evolved to become a miraculous place to live. I've learned that just because the great majority might think I should do something this way or that, does not mean that I am required to abide based on their belief system.

If you have ever been scolded to do something a certain way or told that you should do this or that, remember that you hold all the answers. Your method is right for you. We can still be considerate of the way that other people do things and usually their intention is for good or well-being, but we have all experienced spite or rage against us as people, and when this occurs we do not have to take what they say too seriously, or we end up holding unnecessary resentments against each other.

When I write out a problem for me to resolve or while I write for my books, I try to remember to go slow and take my time. Sometimes the slower, the better. My intention is set to write from a place of clarity and compassion for myself and anyone who ends up reading the material. I try not to feel panicked about getting the words right or rushed. (I'm sure you have heard the story about the tortoise and the hare. In the end, the tortoise won the race due to a tenacious and persevering spirit. There is another saying that goes, "slowly, slowly, catch the monkey." Sometimes the slower we go, the more we achieve.) We must believe in our unique knowledge, abilities, and skills no matter how insignificant we might think they are. I find that belief in our own truth is vital when it comes to writing for resolving personal issues.

When I give myself the opportunity and permit myself to tap into my intuition, my instinct speaks its mind. In fact, a whole new world might appear. I absolutely love to explore whatever rises to the surface!

Interactive Element: Thought Journaling

Activity: Spend 10 minutes each day writing down your thoughts without filtering or judging them. At the end of the week, review your entries and identify any recurring themes or insights about your mental state.

Example: "Each day, I spent ten minutes writing down my unfiltered thoughts. Reviewing my entries at the end of the week, I noticed a recurring theme of self-doubt. Acknowledging these thoughts helped me understand my mental patterns and work towards more positive thinking."

PURPOSE DRIVEN:

It is necessary for humans to feel that life is worth living. If we do not see life as meaningful, useful, or helpful in some way, we lose the motivation to exist and, as a consequence, our happiness and satisfaction. Health tends to gradually deteriorate. Sometimes curiosity leads us to our most profound purpose. Other times, a life purpose drops into our lap, hits us over the head, or we are forced into it, seemingly by accident, but could be by divine plan. Maybe a collective theatre is at play. Life is easier to digest when we are aware of all the components involved in humanity's evolution.

CENTERED FOR LIFE

Love, Peace, and Joy is humanity's natural state, and anything less is caused by forgetting who we are at the core. At the deepest center of our being, we are love, peace, and joy. When I feel the most unlikeable or forgotten, I have found that if I pay attention to my spirit self—the core of who I am, my mood rises, and I trust in my capabilities as a result. We are either filled with spiritual attributes like love, trust, and joy, or hatred, doubt, and fear. Sometimes, yes, life is difficult. In fact, it can be downright impossible some moments. We, humans, have been so smothered by the harshness of earthly experiences. Sometimes the density comes in the form of dwelling and mulling over situations, and it can cause us to go mad. There is a heaviness on this plane of existence, a deep hurt that all humans experience—for the fall of man is the human experience. When we fall, how do we stand back up again? That is the question. Sometimes we must stand again and again, just like toddlers do. This is how we progress, move on, and evolve.

Beliefs that do not align with our authentic self will cause pain and turmoil, so we must really listen to the words and messages we tell ourselves, each moment, every day. (Typically, it's the self-critical thoughts that have to do with assuming that we are not good enough on some level that will sabotage us.) Whenever I suffer or when life seems meaningless, I examine the collection of thoughts that make up my beliefs. Hurtful views are not aligned with the higher universal oneness. Humans have felt this way for years, decades, and centuries—since the beginning of time!

In truth, we are planting seeds. Every little thing we do out of the goodness of our heart is a seed of potential. Each life is a kernel of something great. Just being alive is great! We do not have to be inventive or build something magnificent. We do not have to be number one at anything, and we do not need to try to prove that We Are Right W.A.R. Righteousness perpetuates war. We are not required to explore our inner territory. The way of a fulfilled life is trusting ourselves, the collective community, and the journey of the soul. Just a reminder:

Be Kind to Yourself

Important gifts we can give ourselves are to not only see and appreciate ourselves for who we truly are at our core and all the surface "imperfections" (that come along with the package) but also to love and like who we are and give ourselves concern because as hokey as this might sound, in the end, kindness really does matter. Sometimes spending a few moments focusing on self-consideration can help, but consistent minute-by-minute empathy and compassion for ourselves benefit the most.

In addition to this casual self-care treatment, a more formalized time-out for ourselves can boost our mood and the environment's energy level. A formal session, like an acupressure or a reiki treatment can usually last from forty-five minutes to an hour, depending on preference, the ailment that needs attention, how much time available, and how much concentration we can maintain. For best results, be sure the area we work in is as neat, clean, and comfortable as possible. Avoid tight clothing. Remove shoes, glasses, and jewelry. Wash hands. Lie down in a comfortable position and begin with a receptive mindset that can be recited aloud or to oneself. A number of practices can create an atmosphere of restoration and rejuvenation. We can borrow from the incantation used by Reiki Masters to assist with mindfulness and to place our focus on the here and now, rather than past events.

If you meditate but have dominant thoughts and feelings that seem to interrupt the process, imagine the thoughts as separate from you. Imagine them dissolving or passing by like fluffy white clouds. A cloud does not have the power to destroy the sky. They are here one moment and gone the next.

Does not matter who we are or our origin. Our ancestors utilized foundational tools and progressed through life, relying on what they had on hand, and progress they did! Part of the reason we feel down and out is that we may have forgotten to utilize the natural resources right at our fingertips. Be mindful of your abilities. If you catch yourself worrying or getting angry, picture your energy flowing, free of blockage.

Mindfulness can serve as a moving meditation. Throughout time humanity has diminished the profound significance of the most foundational and fundamental living skills—as if chores are mundane and have little value. As a consequence, the people who take the time and effort to work at hard labor jobs are sometimes the most vilified and demeaned. Mindfulness can also be described as appreciating the work of the least of these and giving all people the highest value. To accomplish difficult tasks, living in the now is a must. Perhaps these individuals are masters at appreciating each moment. Living in the now may sound like a new age concept, but it can be one of the most powerful foundational tools for turning floundering into flourishing—a life with integrity. Doing what's right because it's the right thing to do, not because one will receive a reward for having done so.

To obtain the rewards that we strive for, we must be willing to accept—even love—the most "unacceptable" part of ourselves, and others. This unconditional consideration for all that exists transforms negatives into positives. By being mindful throughout the day, we bring energy to our day-to-day routine. We can utilize mother earth at any time of the day or night to add to a calm, peaceful mind. We can use visualization to create a new future for ourselves—whatever future we wish it to be. When we strive to go back to Zen, our ancient roots open up a portal of endless possibilities. We must accept the hidden aspects of self: our "uncivilized" ancestors. They were smarter than we ever gave them credit for!

Because ancient remedies are natural and non-invasive, there are few risks or side effects. The best results are generated through clean and healthy living. Complementary and alternative therapies transform circumstances from the inside out, and vice versa. You could see a wide range of health benefits appear. When the body is in balance, so too is the mind.

Interactive Element: Balance Exercise

Activity: Practice a balance exercise, such as standing on one leg or using a balance board, for a few minutes each day. Reflect on how physical balance can influence your mental and emotional stability.

Example: "Practicing standing on one leg for a few minutes each day improved my physical balance and also helped me feel more grounded and centered in my daily life. It became a metaphor for finding balance in all aspects of life."

THE LIGHT INVOCATION

"I invoke the light of life within,
I am a clear and perfect channel,
Light is my guide,
I am what I say I am, and
I experience what I say I experience.
In this way, I am paying attention to my energy and creating positive energy."

A Healing Remedy:
To activate the heart chakra, reflect upon the light invocation or the following reiki mantra or any affirmations from your source of inspiration.

"Just for today, I will let go of worry.
Just for today, I will let go of anger.
Just for today,
I give thanks for my many blessings.
Just for today, I will do my work generously.
Just for today,
I will be kind to my neighbors and all living beings."

MOVE TO IMPROVE

Building muscle and strength is not just about aesthetics or athletic performance; it plays a crucial role in enhancing longevity and overall health. As we age, maintaining muscle mass and strength becomes increasingly important for several reasons. Muscle strength is directly linked to functional independence. Strong muscles support daily activities such as lifting, carrying, and even simple movements like standing up from a chair. As we grow older, muscle loss can lead to frailty and a higher risk of falls and injuries. By engaging in regular strength training, we can preserve muscle mass, enhance stability, and maintain our independence well into our later years.

Secondly, muscle health contributes significantly to metabolic health. Muscle tissue is metabolically active, meaning it burns calories even at rest. This helps regulate body weight and prevents obesity-related conditions such as type 2 diabetes and cardiovascular disease. Additionally, strength training improves insulin sensitivity, which is crucial for managing blood sugar levels and reducing the risk of diabetes.

Furthermore, building muscle and strength has profound effects on mental health. Physical activity, including strength training, stimulates the release of endorphins, which are natural mood lifters. Regular exercise can reduce symptoms of depression and anxiety, boost self-esteem, and improve overall mental well-being. As a result, incorporating strength training into your routine can lead to a healthier, happier life.

Small and simple lifestyle changes such as mini-exercises and breathing consciously (deliberately) can improve meditation practice. When I feel better, I tend to have the energy for more activities. The oxygenated and nutrient-enriched brain is able to think clearer and therefore leaves room to see each situation as the new day it is. I also discovered the pain-relieving benefits of minerals.

Eating lean proteins, whole grains, fruits, and vegetables (and less processed foods) are ingredients that provide the body with the fuel needed to motivate me through each day and keep me focused on the tasks at hand. Whole grains and complete proteins level out the blood sugar and decrease cravings for food. The result is sustained energy. Highly-processed foods do not provide the vitamins and minerals my body needs and even prevent the cells from absorbing the necessary nutrients. I drink herbal teas for additional benefits and try to habitually drink a cup of tea in the evening to unwind from a stressful day.

DON'T FORGET TO BALANCE THE MIND WITH PHYSICAL MOVEMENT:

The body is a live vehicle, and like all vehicles, it needs movement or function will eventually decrease. Exercise and movement are essential not only for physical health but also for emotional and mental stamina. Traditional Chinese medicine includes acupuncture, massage, plants and herbs, dietary therapy, and qigong exercises. Shiatsu massage, polarity massage, spiritual healing, Reiki, and other such energy-oriented types of energy therapy can be especially useful in relaxing the nervous system. Circulation prevents body imbalances and stagnation.

Hydration is central to keeping our bodily systems working optimally. The human body is composed mostly of water and required to flush out impurities that add up from daily processes. Proper hydration sustains the energy level, and

where to find peace so you can live like mad

aids in burning the fuel taken in by way of food. I found that soda with lunch made me feel tired and sluggish for the rest of the day, so I slowly made the change to drink more and more water throughout the day instead of sugary drinks. (I still enjoy drinking at least one cup of coffee in the morning, but I try to drink more water, and I found that I am better energized.)

> **DEEP CONSCIOUS BREATHING** is crucial for the copious flow of life force throughout the body and to oxygenate the brain. Bio-energy is the source of all activity and manifestation. Tactical breathing throughout the day increases energy levels and keeps us humans balanced and harmonious. We will be less prone to low emotional states or illness.

Add movement to the schedule: Our bodies only burn so many calories daily. This can be fulfilled by simply taking a pleasurable one-mile walk during lunch or after work. I know I could definitely do better in this department. (This is a great time for self-coaching using positive self-talk.) Keep the body active on a daily basis. Self-care aids in the vitality needed to be more productive at home or work and raises our mood.

GOING BACK TO ZEN

It is human nature to tell ourselves that we will wait until something happens before we can be happy. Most times it's about having more money, or a more enjoyable job, or once we finish our schooling, then we can relax. Waiting for something to happen before we allow ourselves to be fully happy can easily become habitual. Before we know it, we might say we can only be happy after we reach retirement. The secret, according to Tao (The Way of Nature), is to be rooted in our sacred energy life force (S.E.L.F.) along the path—even when it is a struggle, or it seems as if others have more than us—life is then simplified. Thus, happiness is not contingent on external happenings, or we would be waiting a long time. Simplicity becomes the way!

> **MOVEMENT** strengthens the muscles and nerves and therefore rejuvenates the body and the mind when we need to be alert and proactive. Exercise contributes to the development of a sturdy and healthy immune system serving as a time to restore and recover from daily stress.

Of course, certain thoughts will interrupt our peace, but we have the ability to acknowledge them. Most suffering is caused by resistance against the reality of the situation. Yes, those closest to us, and those not so close, will astound and disappoint us, but to expect that everyone read their moral compassion and thus make choices accordingly will only disappoint us further. When what is isn't fair, we have the right to examine further and disagree, to voice our point of view and put forth our opinion. The earth terrain can be harsh! Expect that we will be hit with resistance—and the resistance isn't so shocking to our systems.

For holistic and healthy living, I try to listen to what my cells are telling me. If something doesn't feel right, it is the body's way of saying pay attention to a certain area. Maybe it is time to visit a doctor, to do some of my own research, or to move a little more than usual. When I make a few small changes, I change the course of my biology and history—and this has an impact on others and alters the future. Listening is a great way to discover what needs to be done, how to do it, and when to start. This is the reason I am a fan of "isolation." A few moments of silence or even a long time in isolation can really put troubling circumstances into perspective and help us to discover what in life is most important.

Investing time in building muscle and strength is an investment in your future health and longevity. By incorporating regular strength training exercises into your schedule, you can enhance your physical capabilities, support your metabolic health, and improve your mental well-being, ensuring a more vibrant and independent life as you age.

Interactive Element: Add Movement to Your Schedule

Activity: Create a small exercise space in your home with motivational elements. Use this space for daily exercise for building or maintaining strength. Document how this dedicated space helps you feel energized. Or schedule in time to take a walk either in the morning or evening.

GOING BACK TO ZEN

Example: "I created a small workout space in my garage with a few motivational posters and an exercise chart to keep me on track and excited. Making time for movement brought a sense of empowerment and health to my life and health is wealth.

TAP INTO YOUR INTUITION

Throughout the centuries, people all over the world have used meditation to transform their lives. They have used it to improve their health and to better manage their emotions. Making time for self can change one's life.

Most of all, isolation gifts us time to de-clutter the brain for better decision making. We gain a more clarified perspective on the soul's point of view. We become more aware of what's going on in life and better able to decide if we should stay on course or make necessary changes. If you have ever been accused of being a loner, take it as a compliment. Maybe this time was meant to be, or time alone serves a meaningful purpose. It does not mean tomorrow will be the same—it just means for now. All of life is temporary. However, when we use isolation to avoid feelings of rejection, this is when we need to take courageous steps to trust that everyone is going through something and risk being rejected if it means attaining potential purpose. Life is vulnerable, and all humans have the challenge of somehow surviving. It does not matter how perfect appearances are, everyone is faced with suffering at one time or another.

Meditation inspires humanity to become more loving and compassionate towards self and others. If you're one of the many people who have the tendency to put yourself down and you want to change the way you have been treating yourself, self-awareness can slow down and stop thoughts on autopilot and assist you in becoming more alert of a potentially abusive inner dialogue. When we recognize how we talk to ourselves, and if we find that we say unkind things, we can then give ourselves more consideration and appreciation.

Strong emotions such as anger, fear, and even jealousy can be managed when we are willing to see from the perspective of others. When we meditate, we choose authenticity—that does not mean that we have to ignore or repress judgmental feelings. On the contrary, authenticity is honesty. It's about realizing that all are human. This allows us to tackle real feelings without shame or judgment toward self or others. Confronting heartfelt feelings allows for the truth to rise to the surface (even when the mainstream disagrees with us) so that we can hear the genuineness of self, thus know the inner self better, accept self as is, and free self from any uneasy and disruptive feelings.

Authenticity also improves relationships. From a receptive mode, we better understand the larger circumstances surrounding the topic and are therefore aware of the well-meaning intent or just plain humanness of others. We become active listeners, better able to control judgmental thoughts because we no longer see others through the fearful egoic lens that paints everyone else as wrong and ourselves as right. We give others the freedom to be who they are, to believe what they want to believe, and accept imperfections without burdening them with expectations, wants, and needs. It helps us to manage the ego.

Silence improves our attunement with our logic, instincts, and intuition. Listening assists us to be clear about our own life purpose, aligning with the genuine path specified for each individual. That way, we won't be overwhelmed by thinking of all the things we need to do or try to do things all at once. It helps us have a laser-like focus that can cut through steel. While we do things one at a time, we are able to finish our work faster, no longer distracted by intrusive thoughts.

Authenticity found from tapping into our intuition pushes worry out of the way. Worrying is dwelling on the worst-case scenarios. In contrast, listening to the true self places the focus on the present moment, abilities, solutions, and offers peace to potential problems. By staying relaxed and in tune with the present, we exercise willpower over the future.

We are able to look at each situation without falling for the assumption that we are guilty of wanting to revert back to our own nature. When we accept life as it is, it is then that we can adapt or make the necessary changes for the betterment of all involved. Making changes is easier when on the path of least resistance and not full of expectations. This does not mean ignoring human rights violations or crimes. It means when we are faced with problems, we acknowledge that the path we are on is not working. How do we know? The path could be causing discomfort, or it is our beliefs about the path that is causing turmoil. We are then able to investigate the issue from as many sides as possible, and after considering all possible solutions, we can discern which thoughts and beliefs need to change. Time alone gives us the space to clear our minds so that we can see from a neutral perspective. From a calm mind, light bulb solutions pop up.

Interactive Element: Intuition Journal

Activity: Keep a journal where you record intuitive insights or gut feelings. Reflect on these entries and note any patterns or how often your intuition guides you correctly. Keep in mind that sometimes untrue beliefs or assumptions about certain situations or people can cause us to experience feelings that are not true and will sabotage our well being and relationships.

Example: "I kept a journal of intuitive insights and gut feelings. Reviewing my entries, I noticed that my intuition was often

where to find peace so you can live like mad

correct, especially regarding decisions at work. This practice boosted my confidence in trusting my inner voice."

STOP AND SMELL THE FLOWERS

Upon my older daughter's high school graduation, we visited the lavender farms in Sequim, Washington, and fell in love with the scent of the purple blooms. We bought soaps, lotions, teas, sachets, and a scented stuffed pillow, which could be heated for tummy aches. We even tried the lavender ice cream! My curiosity on the topic thereafter led me to the uses of the floral essence. I learned that lavender can assist the brain waves in flowing smoothly, producing an increase in restful alpha waves seated at the back region of the brain. (Jasmine targets the alert and aware beta waves located at the front of the brain.) I believe the aroma gently anchored my daughter into ease and comfort while she adapted to her first year in college and dorm life. Other benefits from the lavender include relaxing and clarifying the mind for studying. My daughter graduated and is now a teacher. A little aromatherapy has proven to be far-reaching for our family!

A French chemist by the name of René-Maurice Gattefossé burned his hand during an experiment in a perfumery plant a little more than one hundred years ago. Because he could not find an immediate remedy, he plunged his hand into a vat of lavender essential oil to stop the burning. It is rumored that his hand miraculously recovered, and later the researcher discovered the ointment ceased infection and left no visible scarring. Gattefossé concluded that the plant-based essential oil could heal, and started to experiment with more botanicals. He originated the term Aromatherapy in the first published book on the topic, titled Gattefosse's Aromatherapy. When another French doctor ran out of antibiotics during World War II, he turned to Gattefosse's studies on the oils to treat gangrene and wounds, and then went on to write The Practice of Aromatherapy: A Classic Compendium of Plant Medicines and Their Healing Properties. Aromatherapy soon became acceptable in Western culture. The rest is modern history!

Essential oils can be inhaled by a diffuser, applied topically, and even available in dietary supplements. Aromatic oils are distilled by a steam process, or cold-pressed from bark, trees, flowers, and herbs, and the practice goes back for more than 6000 years in the African continent, India, China, Egypt, Rome, and Greece. (While growing up, you may have heard the Bible tale mentioning three wise men from the east who brought gifts of gold, frankincense, and myrrh to the young parents of Yeshua [Ancient Aramaic].[4]

Apart from being used as a fragrance, frankincense oil of the African genus Boswellia tree (originally from Somalia, Oman, and Yemen) has numerous medicinal uses. Sadly, the tree is endangered and could disappear in about fifty years due to exploitation. More than 82% of the product comes from Somalia, with some frankincense also gathered in adjacent Southern Arabia and Ethiopia, Sudan, and other central African countries.

---

4. Jesus, otherwise known as Issa [Arabic] or Isa in Islam and in some parts of the Middle East and Asia, is referred to as Jesus in English/Christianity. The name "Isa" is commonly used in Arabic-speaking and Islamic contexts, with the Quran mentioning Isa (Jesus) multiple times, emphasizing his prophetic role. This reflects the influence of Islamic culture and language in these regions. In English, the name "Jesus" is derived from the Greek "Iēsous," which comes from the Hebrew "Yeshua." This name is used widely in Christian traditions and is documented throughout the Bible. By exploring these cultural and religious contexts, we can understand the different names and titles used for Jesus across various regions, religions and belief systems.

GOING BACK TO ZEN

The tree itself looks like an aged miracle. Its oil wields an antiseptic that can be applied to wounds to eliminate germs without the side effects. The oil has also been used to reduce scars, promote digestion, and take care of mouth sores, toothaches, and infections. Myrrh, another "baby shower" gift given to Yeshua's parents, is a resin or sap-like substance, also common in Africa and the Middle East. The myrrh tree is unique due to its knotted and aged-trunk. Oils from this tree boost the immune system along with countless more advantages.

Aromatherapy is a treatment that also uses extracted plant oils through massaging or inhalation. The Egyptians are believed to have invented the early oil distillation device. The antibacterial remedy delivers a healing solution dating back thousands of years over the Americas. Native Americans used nutmeg oils to ward off intestine problems. Aromatherapy can uplift or relax, introduce a romantic flair into the air, and relief from aching muscles.

Evidence also indicates that distillment plays a significant part of the culture in India. The practice of Ayurveda comprises a myriad of uses from nature's bounty. In addition to incorporating flavor and aroma into meals, plants have been traditionally used to treat diseases. India's rich tradition has optimized the applications of spices into food and beverages like teas. The curative results are well-documented in their system of preventive medicine.

> Remember, after hard falls and deep winters, spring always arrives.

Let's savor every moment we have alive and remember the perceptions we hold, and the words we use to describe ourselves and others really do matter. Sometimes it's the hardships that prompt us to dig down deep and find our value and our strength to look at life from a renewed, more

where to find peace so you can live like mad

appreciative perspective. Don't fear the speed bumps, hurdles, stumbling blocks, and great walls for they can be the starting point from which we can evolve and grow to become the persistent and prevailing humans we were born to be. Always remember you are rooted in an invisible and everlasting force, deeper and wider than ever imagined.

***

I'll always remember the time my younger high school-aged daughter and I were doing laps around the track and field. She had just begun a photography hobby. We were deep in conversation (well, maybe, I was doing most of the talking) when all of a sudden, she put her fingers to her lips and shushed me. Shhh. She told me, "Be quiet!" She had spotted something! Of course, I had to ask, "what do you see?" She yelped, "A dandelion!" and then ran toward the thing for a photography session. My lesson for the day? Dandelions are not just ugly weeds that intrude upon our back and front yard spaces, they can be seen as brilliant blooms of sunlight taking up residence on maintained lawns, golf courses, in the corners of brick buildings, and even breaking through the crevices of cement walkways.

This Eurasian flower, seen and treated as an unwanted weed to most of us westerners, is believed to have survived and evolved from about 30 million years. Have you noticed that these lowly yellow blooms can even rise and break through sidewalks and buckle cement? It's because, like all of nature, their roots run deep and long and everlasting. Yes, they are hated by many of us. But, sometimes, when the world turns upside down, it's time for us to take a look at life from the bottom up. Only then can we find valuables beneath the surface and rise to a new occasion.

Mother Nature has provided so much more for us to stop and appreciate. All we need to do is be willing to see from a different angle. Maybe from the ground up rather than from the top down. We can enjoy the scents of nature in our very own yards, peeking out from the most unlikely raggedy places. Let's reap the results!

(Who would have thought this weed could be beneficial?) Most commonly, it is sold in tea packs at grocery marts, but some people have made a dandelion coffee, and even wine, and we can also purchase freshly bundled dandelion greens at health food stores for salads and whatnot, or capsules from vitamin shops. (Personally, I'm too afraid to transform it into a mealtime lunch. Doesn't sound so appealing. I have yet to cook with it. ;-))

Rich in vitamin C and Luteolin (a flavonoid compound found in fruits and vegetables), it has been used to protect the bones from age-related damage, improving overall bone health. It's also used in various parts of the world to treat liver disorders, control diabetes, urinary issues, acne, cancer, and so on. And yes, this is crazy, you can eat every single part of the dandelion. (Just don't sit on your front lawn and stuff flowers in your mouth! Your neighbors will think you've really gone mad!)

Besides its little round pocket of yellow sunshine, dandelion offers a plethora of medicinal benefits just like other plants. Did you know the dandelion, which translates into "lion's tooth," is rich in calcium, iron, and vitamins A and C? (I'm still too afraid to try any from my neck of the woods. Eek. Lol.)

Sometimes when we are forced to see from the ground up (or the back alley), we are led to a healthy, transformational, and fulfilling life. Sometimes life's most difficult challenges are the seeds that guide us to our true purpose. Through the process of navigation, and given the opportunity to claim our authentic power, we become the person we were born to be. This evolution has led me to revert back to my ethnic roots and recoup all that it provides.

Like the dandelion flower, have you ever felt misunderstood, labeled, reduced down to a caricature, perceived as someone you're not, or was forced to deal with an unexpected and drastic change? Perhaps, this is the human experience. Maybe all of us have felt this way. After all is said and done, one thing remains, we are much more than we ever thought we were! We are connected to all that is! Let's get up and escape from stress, worry, and anxiety. We can hit the reset button and begin again if need be.

For the times you are hit with surprising news—news that turns your world upside, let's get down close to the earth and stop to smell the flowers—err, I mean, whatever we can. Doesn't mean we have to eat everything we see, but just an FYI: according to Mother Nature, nothing is off-limits.

The civilized world can feel harsh and unwelcoming at times, and every so often we get so caught up in the business of ordinary life we forget about our earth mother's true nature. When we live close to the land, the wonders from it can offer us a renewed perspective, and uplift us. Sometimes lighting a few scented candles and listening to just the right music (whatever music you enjoy) can set the right mood to decompress from a tense environment invoking well-being, confidence, and receptivity for all those nearby.

And... along the way, stop and smell the roses—or lavender—or any flower—or hug a tree or pick a dandelion—whatever suits your fancy!

Interactive Element: Nature Journaling

Activity: Spend time observing a natural setting (a park, garden, or even a potted plant). Choose a flower or plant and observe it closely. Notice its colors, shapes, and any scents. Reflect on how this mindfulness practice affects your stress levels and mental clarity. Write a journal entry about your observations and how connecting with nature impacts your sense of peace.

Example: "I spent a few minutes closely observing roses in my garden. Noticing their vibrant colors, delicate petals, and subtle fragrance, I felt a deep appreciation for their beauty. I wrote about the different colors, the sound of birds, and the feel of the breeze. This mindful practice calmed my mind, heightened my awareness of nature's beauty and brought a profound sense of connection, enriching my day."

MORE FROM MOTHER NATURE'S BOUNTY

These are just a few examples of endless gifts nature consistently provides and offered here as ideas to investigate if you so wish. Two of my favorite on-hand resource books are The Complete Guide to Herbal Medicines by Charles W. Fetrow Pharm.D. and Juan R. Avila, PharmD and The Green Pharmacy by James A. Duke, Ph.D.. Also, while my daughters were growing up, I liked to have the Encyclopedia of Natural Medicine by Michael Murray, N.D., and Joseph Pizzorno, N.D., close at hand just in case we encountered a non-medical emergency or simply curious.

> They tried to bury us.
>
> They didn't know we were seeds.
>
> Mexican Proverb

- **African Bluegrass** is in the same family as lemongrass and citronella and used as an astringent, antifungal agent, antiviral agent, and is prepared to be massaged into feet. The medium scented blend has a hint of floral and citrus notes.

For a "holy" blend, combine the African bluegrass oil with the oils of citronella, olive, and myrrh.

- Another not as well-known citus is **Bergamot,** found in South East Asian lands, Europe, and the Mediterranean. The sweet aroma oil of bergamot comes from the lumpy bulbous peels of the lime-like fruit used to mitigate stress, fatigue, arthritis, bronchitis, water retention, migraines, nervousness, and skin infections. The Asian-based spiny citrus tree grows sour pear-shaped fruits used to produce perfumes.
- **Cedarwood Atlas** comes from plants, rather than wood, to uplift the spirit, tone the skin, and ground the soul. The wood comes from cedar, a member of the juniper family, and has been used by the Egyptians for spiritual embalming purposes.
- **Chamomile** can be found in tea form in grocery stores and has a reputation for calming one's mood. Also, as a solution used to relieve joint inflammation and arthritic symptoms, the herb is said to address numerous things such as cuts, headaches, boils, insomnia, skin irritations, sunburns, dry skin, eczema and insect bites. Among other benefits, Chamomile tea treats gastrointestinal issues and reduces belly bloating.
- **Cinnamon bark** has a robust fragrance compared to the leaf variant and wards against colds, flu, chills, and related illnesses. It is one of the most common spices for flavoring and found predominantly in many cultures, including Ayurvedic medicine. Cinnamon is also used for slowing contractions or cramps, yeast infections, arthritis, and digestive problems. Among so many advantages, the oil can heal bee stings, reduce stress, control blood sugar levels, and boost brain function!
- **Citrus,** such as lemons, limes, clementines, and grapefruit, revitalize the body and contains astringent properties that aid in clearing up oily skin. Citrus has a fresh and invigorating scent known to uplift the spirit and relieve insomnia while producing a refreshing sensation. Sometimes my husband will use citrus to clean his fingers if we are out and about, but without access to water.

GOING BACK TO ZEN

- **According** to those who use **Cypress French oils** distilled from the needle-bearing conifer tree, the claim is that the primary benefit is associated with contraction. Cypress oil tightens muscles and hair follicles, which prevents teeth and hair from falling out. It is also used for treating external and internal wounds and tones the respiratory system. The spicy, masculine fragrance makes a great natural smelling deodorant.
- **Eucalyptus** is a botanic Latin-based oil extracted from wood and leaves. The tall and beautiful trees are adorned with tough leaves, and clusters of amazing looking red or white buds surrounded by what appear to be tassels. The tree includes properties to treat skin illness, such as blisters, insect bites, burns, skin infections, wounds, colds, and flu. Eucalyptus oils purify, cool, balance, and revitalize the body and mind. Peppermint oils invigorate, refresh, and cool, promoting energy. During allergy season, I like to place a smudge under my nose. (In other words, I'm "smearing" myself. — That is a joke!) This way, I don't bother others around me with my personal choice of perfume. One of my favorite scents to wash my hands with is citrus, like lemon or grapefruit.
- **Nutmeg Essential Oil** has a warm, sweet, woody scent. It is similar to the cooking spice, but richer and more fragrant. Egyptians used nutmeg as part of the embalming process. In the Middle Ages, nutmeg was grated and mixed with lard as an ointment for hemorrhoids. Nutmeg is a potent warming oil, and in very small quantities can help to revitalize and warm soreness and circulation.
- **Rosemary** boosts memory, relieves pain, and protects the immune system from bacterial infections. Try dicing up the evergreen needles into olive oil and lemon, then dipping garlic bread into the mix. Like Rosemary, oregano can help with treating a congested respiratory tract. In fact, I've overheard my Filipino and Vietnamese neighbors mention oregano in a potted plant can be used any time to strengthen the immunity against bacteria and viruses. Whenever they feel a sore throat, cold, or flu coming on, they snip a little herb to cook with or use for teas. This herb, which means

"delight of the mountains," also can be used to remedy nail fungus and deter lice, bed bugs, mosquitoes, and fleas. And, like rosemary, oregano can be used to treat fungal infections like athlete's foot. Try a footbath at the end of the day!

We are fortunate today to have easy access to scented candles, lotions, soaps, potpourri, perfumes, colognes, and reed diffusers. The aromatic extracts soothe the body and mind and lessen our burdens from a variety of ailments thrown at us by the "civilized" world. Above is a short list I've gathered of earthly treasures from nature's bounty, maybe already found all around you.

Interactive Element: Foraging Walk

Activity: Take a guided foraging walk (in person or virtually) to learn about edible and medicinal plants in your area. Document what you learn and how this knowledge enhances your connection to nature.

Example: "During a guided foraging walk, I learned to identify edible plants like mint and wild garlic. Once home, I washed the mint leaves thoroughly and prepared a refreshing mint tea by boiling water and pouring it over a handful of fresh mint leaves. I let it steep for 5 - 10 minutes and then strained the tea and sweetened with honey. This experience deepened my connection to nature and inspired me to incorporate foraged ingredients into my meals."

CONCLUSION: GOING FROM RICHES TO RAGS

Once upon a time, there lived a prince who was protected by the grand walls of a royal palace. This prince was unlike the others as he wanted to live a simple life lacking what everyone else wished for and wanted. His father, the king of the palace, surrounded his son with only beautiful beings—things that were pleasing to the eye and would satisfy the prince.

During the boy's childhood, the prince enjoyed all the spoils of a comfortable life. He grew to master the traditional arts and sciences of his time and culture without needing instruction. It is rumored that he learned numerous languages and was skilled at mathematics without much study. He also became proficient at sports such as martial arts and archery.

The king's biggest fear was that his son would be touched by the pain of others, and this would cause the young man grief. So the king focused on protecting and securing his son from the knowledge of mortality and death. He kept his son within the palace walls to prevent him from witnessing the sorrows of the outside world, but the prince's curiosity led him to wonder what was outside the kingdom despite his father's resolve.

To prevent unnecessary distress on his son, the king ordered the palace walls to be high enough to shield the boy from the dangers and sadness of the outside world. This lasted until his son's teen years, but eventually, the prince matured, his curiosity intensified, and this prompted his desire to look beyond the palace's imperial gates. He begged his father to allow him outside, but the king was afraid that his son would be unable to cope with the realities of the outliers. (And why would a prince want to go outside when everything he could ever want was inside the walls? After all, his father had given him anything and everything he could ever wish for.)

The prince was so insistent that the king reluctantly relented at last, but he arranged for his son only planned excursions. The king tried to remove the aged, suffering and deceased from his son's view, and instead fill the outside community immediately beyond the gates with lovely sights. He had the attendants shoo away anyone or anything that appeared sickly and replaced the citizens with beautiful and attractive people and positive things for the prince to look at as he rode along by chariot.

And by chariot, the prince left the premises chaperoned by an aide to answer questions as they drove on a gilded path embellished with fragrant and lovely flowers through the community. Finally, outside of the protection of his father's kingdom, the prince saw many unusual things stirring his longing to experience more. He felt compelled to explore. The first time out of the walled gates, the prince spotted an elder man hobbling along. He asked, "What is that creature stumbling, shabby, bent, and broken beside my retinue"?

His assistant answered, "That is a man, like other men, who was born an infant, became a child, a youth; he has been a father, a father of fathers. This man has become old, subject to destruction of his beauty, his will, and the possibilities of life, like other men."

"That means this will happen to me?" asked the prince. The attendant replied, "Inevitably with the passage of time.'"

The king's staging backfired. It didn't matter how much he tried to make life appear perfect; whatever he excluded came out of the woodworks and haunted the king's wish for refinement and perfection.

The prince returned to the kingdom devastated from learning that life ages and eventually declines. It took him many months to recover from what felt like one of the biggest lies. Life isn't all roses and butterflies. Life eventually devolves.

After months of recovering from post-traumatic stress disorder, the prince ventured out again, still recuperating from the aging world outside his own.

The second time outside of the kingdom, he noticed an ill man at the side of the royal path. "This creature," he asked, "shaking and palsy-afflicted, unbearable to behold a source of pity in contempt, what is he?"

And was told, "That's a man like other men who were born whole but who became ill and sick and unable to cope; a burden to himself and others, suffering and incurable, like other men."

"You say," the prince asked, astounded at the thought, "and this could happen to me?"

"No man is exempt from the ravages of disease," said the assistant.

Again, the prince needed time to convalesce after learning such bitter truth.

The third time beyond the palace walls, the young prince noticed a funeral processional. A corpse laid out before him. He wanted to know what it was. The attendant said, "That is a man like other men. Born, beloved and hated, who was once like you, and now the earth, like other men."

"You say, then," the prince asked, "this could happen to me?"

"This is your end and the end of all men," answered his aide.

The prince returned home, devastated at the thought. He had trouble forgetting the images of the human condition. Even though the king tried to shield his son from the realities of life, the son was destined to face reality sooner or later—because that is what life requires. Similarly to how our arm or leg might tingle (painfully) after awakening from lying on it wrong, the awareness of suffering might be painful at first, and it might take time to recover. We will fall and fail as we try to wobble to a standing position.

where to find peace so you can live like mad

Witnessing suffering left a deep impression on the prince's mind and led him to realize that all living beings without exception have to be experienced: the pains of birth, sickness, aging, and death. Because the prince understood the laws of reincarnation, he also realized that humans experience these sufferings not just once, but again and again, in life after life without cessation. Seeing living beings trapped in this vicious circle of grief, he developed a sincere wish to free all of humanity from grief and pain.

The realization that he, like anyone else, could be subject to different forms of human turmoil drove the man into a personal crisis.

He resolved to leave the palace once and for all, and engage in contemplation. He hoped that knowledge gained from meditation and reflection would lead to liberation (and salvation) from burdensome emotional pain. But, his father stubbornly feared to allow his son to leave the safety of the kingdom. The king wanted his son to only know extravagant privileges and the positive life the king could afford his son.

But Prince Siddhartha contested his father's protection. The young man came up with a plan to deprive himself of material possessions, compelled to comprehend the truth of the world around him. He said to his father, "If you can give me permanent freedom from the sufferings of birth, sickness, aging, and death, I shall stay in the palace, but if you cannot, I must leave and make my human life meaningful." Shocked and scared to learn the prince intended to renounce his title and leave the posh premises, the king forcefully denied his son's wish. The king replenished the palace grounds and surroundings with a retinue of beautiful female dancers, singers, and musicians and posted guards around the palace walls. Yet the social events failed. With the help of a trusted aide, the prince made his escape from the palace walls. He even cut off his hair and ordained himself a monk. By the time he was 29, he had abandoned palace life completely and began to live as a homeless ascetic.

He developed a contingency plan for overcoming pain: 1. Suffering exists. (Shocking!) 2. There is a cause of this suffering. (And no one wants to know about the weak or the poor.) 3. There is an end to suffering. (Tune into sacred energy.) 4. The end of suffering can be found in the Eightfold Path. (Natural self.)

Buddha's conclusion? By going back to Zen—otherwise known as the simplicity of life—one can find liberation. He is known for saying, "That is the ancient path, the ancient road, traveled by the rightly self-awakened ones of former times. I followed that path. Following it, I came to direct knowledge of aging and death, direct knowledge of the origination of aging and death, direct knowledge of the cessation of aging and death, direct knowledge of the path leading to the cessation of aging and death. I followed that path. Following it, I came to direct knowledge of birth... becoming... clinging... craving... feeling... contact... direct knowledge of the origin of consciousness, direct knowledge of the cessation of consciousness, direct knowledge of the path leading to the cessation of consciousness. I followed that path." Through the force of sacred energy life force, an enlightened one knows that nothing is permanent. Therefore, an awakened one spontaneously does whatever is appropriate to benefit humanity. This is the Noble Path. It does not matter which path you choose, what matters is how you choose to walk. If the path turns ugly, start exploring it without criticism, but rather with receptive and interested eyes. Rebrand the challenges as a curious new adventure.

You may have heard of the prince. Today he is known as the Buddha, previously Siddhartha Gautama. Buddhist philosophy is now known all over the world. A Buddha is directly and simultaneously aware of his alignment with nature, the universal oneness of all-that-is, and because of this connection with the Source (Taoists sometimes call this the Universal Mother)—the unmanifested—and acknowledgment, he was able to share compassionate ideas and methodology for humanity, embracing the imperfections of life without discrimination to those who suffered beyond his time and space.

Interactive Element: Awareness Practice

Activity: Write down the names of the people you have trouble valuing. Despite their imperfections and annoyances, acknowledge that they also suffer just like all of humanity. All people face difficulties and challenges. Reflect on how this practice affects your overall sense of peace and understanding.

Example: "Each of us has a personal relationship with the universe. Whether or not we adhere to any particular religion, it feels good to cultivate a friendly relationship with the whole of humanity and of nature. We belong to a community of souls who are trying the best they can based on the information they believe in.

AUTHENTICITY:

Each of us has a personal relationship with the universe. Whether or not we adhere to any particular religion, it feels good to cultivate a friendly relationship with the whole of humanity and of nature. We belong to a community of like-minded souls.

GIFT MEDITATION

Many years ago, I realized that pop (aka soda) was making me drowsy and feeling heavy, so I wrote the following passage for myself to increase my water intake. Since then, I have fallen in love with drinking water. The use of my imagination comes in handy when I want to refresh myself with the benefits of drinking water. I thought this would be a nice place to share it with you.

Just a FYI: During meditation, you are in a state of alert receptivity. Your subconscious is in total control. Guided meditations use the power of your imagination and relaxation to develop a rapport with the everlasting part of you. The guided meditation directs your mind to a comfortable place, and then you take yourself to a place of empowerment and peace. You are in charge at all times. **Drink to Your Health! Here's my personal meditation for drinking water.**

Ready? Let's get comfy. Begin by closing your eyes. Let's go to a different time and place. ....Now imagine yourself. ....Now imagine yourself climbing into a small space capsule. You find the most comfortable seat you've ever seen in front of you.

When you sit on the low couch, you sink your legs and back into its restful soft cushions. This protected place is your home away from home. You can feel the plush pillows all around you. You lean back into them, and you feel so content. Nothing can hurt you here. You hear the soft whirl of the space capsule in the background, and it makes you feel even more secure. As you listen to the soothing hum, you relax even more and find a perfect position.

You feel wholly nurtured and protected, knowing that you are closer and closer to your infinite and more aware self. You sense the universal sacred energy life-force all around, and it's the most beautiful thing you've ever felt. You even become aware of the stars gently shooting past you. They look so splendid, as they leave a trail of many strands of glittery light. You feel content and excited about this fantastic adventure—it is an adventure that you control.

You are embraced by the loving energy of the stars. The silence increases your ability to understand the sacred beauty of life that is within every human being. You are enveloped by a sensation of peaceful stillness. You get to decide when to slow down. You decide to gently turn off the engine and savor the warm feeling of this comfortable cocoon.

Imagine yourself filling up a glass with clean, fresh filtered water. Take a second to appreciate the clear and sparkling liquid in the transparent glass. You can see that it is clean and filtered. It looks so refreshing. Now take a sip and savor the cool, reviving clear water. Feel the cool liquid soothe and refresh your tongue, stream around your gums, along with your teeth, and cool your entire mouth. Notice the uplifting, clean water makes its way to energize your body, assisting with its ability to restore itself.

Take another sip and imagine the pure, reviving clear liquid, cleansing your soul. It feels so good. The energizing liquid soothes and refreshes your tongue, streams around your gums, along your teeth, and cools your entire mouth. Notice the water energizing your spirit, assisting with your body's ability to restore itself. Imagine this when you feel tired or as many times as you would like.

You know that you are taking care of your body, keeping it healthy and vivacious. You choose to drink clear, clean water because it suits your needs. You drink water because it keeps you upbeat and healthy. You are a healthy individual, and you love to take care of yourself. Your first choice is to make sure you get enough water in your system every day. Your mind feels free and clear when doing so.

Now spend the next few minutes (or however you long you wish to) to meditate upon this wonderful feeling of healthy living. Whenever you need to feel energized and strengthened, you can turn to water for survival, refreshment, and even refinement. Mother Nature provides without asking for anything in return.

DEAR GENTLE AND WISE SOUL

I wanted to reach out and remind you that you are not alone. I know that you have been struggling with challenges and burdens, and I want you to know that you are loved.

Life's winters can be overwhelming and make it hard to see the good things in life, but please remember that there is hope—spring is around the corner. You are a strong and resilient person, and I believe in your sacred energy life force —the essence of you.

Remember, it's important to give yourself time and space to heal and there are fellow souls allies who care about you and want to support you — you might not see them now or know of their existence. There are also others who could benefit from the optimism, skills, talents, knowledge that you already have within but haven't yet shared to the fullest of your ability.

You have so much to offer the world, and you have already accomplished so much. So many around you are waiting to see all the amazing things you will share. Remember that you are worthy of love and respect, and that your life has meaning and purpose.

If you ever need more tools, reach within yourself for answers. You have a special light within that has the power to brighten the lives of those around you. Listen to those around you for they may need your affection and compassion, your skills and talents.

Coping with human surprises, tragedies, losses, assumptions made against you, and suffering can be difficult and overwhelming. You may not realize this but you have been an inspiration for others. By staying aligned with your greater self, you become an light for others. If they need additional upliftment, below are a few more tips that you can share to pass the torch forward.

Practice self-care: Help yourself and others to find interests that each find enjoyable and relaxing, such as moving, meditation, or spending time in nature. Caring about the emotional and mental well being of all of humanity, motivates all of us to balance our lives with play, work, and rest.

Reach out to others: Talk about emotions can help everyone process what they're going through and provide a sense of understanding and empathy. Be an understanding listening ear for them. It will also benefit you.

Encourage fellow souls to acknowledge their emotions: It's okay to feel sad, angry, or overwhelmed in the face of losses, tragedy or suffering. By recognizing and acknowledging feelings, can help our friends to loosen and release the tied-up emotional knots. Your kind words can uplift and energize not only the person you're reaching out to, but also back to you.

Remember that coping with life —and all that comes with it, including the suffering and tragedies, is a process that takes time. Remind your friends, frenemies and enemies to be patient and kind to themselves and others as they work through their thoughts and find ways to cope with the sufferings of the world.

No one is alone in this journey called life even though it feels like it at times and neither are you. If you are feeling overwhelmed, take time out to rest and reset. It's okay to take a break from the noise.

Remember that you are a strong and resilient person. Believe in your ability and ingenuity to survive and thrive and to help others to do the same. Take care of yourself, and remember that better days are ahead.

With warm regards,

Janine Vance

Author of *The Power of Isolation: How Silence is Golden*

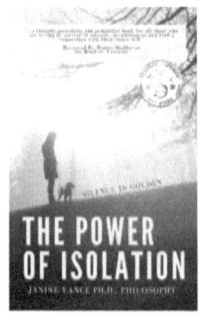

*Additional meditations can be found in *The Power of Isolation: How Silence is Golden*. About the book and a sample chapter are provided in the following pages.

EXCERPT FROM THE POWER OF ISOLATION

This chapter discusses the inevitability of feeling isolated and left out at times. It emphasizes the importance of using these moments of solitude to one's advantage. The chapter encourages you to embrace silence and view it as an opportunity for self-reflection and rejuvenation. By quieting the mind, one can accomplish personal goals and connect with your true self.

Theme: *A Journey of Caregiving and Isolation*

Idea: *View silence as a peaceful friend who brings gifts of clarity and insight*

In my late twenties, despite what seemed like a normal life, I often found it hard to get out of bed and face the day. There was a heaviness that weighed me down. Even though I understood that I was a soul having a human experience, like all humans, there seemed to be something missing. I craved peace and the simple joy of feeling good, but the more I tried to achieve this, the more elusive it became.

It was the year 1984 when my dad, an active and busy engineer, survived a 100-foot hang gliding fall. Our lives changed drastically due to the accident when the wings of the hang glider collapsed in midair and Dad fell into and through a mountain range of large Washington state fir trees. This was when my family's life turned upside down. The accident left him physically disabled and a traumatic brain injury to recover from. I was twelve at the time.

By my twenties, my mother had already passed away from cancer. My husband and I moved Dad in with us, and I quit my job at the beauty salon to be home with him and ensure his care. It was actually convenient for me because I had two young daughters at the time. I could be home with my girls while they were young and all through their high school years. I was very fortunate to be able to do that.

During the 25 years of his life while he lived with me, there were days when the effort to do the simplest tasks felt overwhelming but we made the best of it. Sometimes even getting out of bed and walking up the neighborhood hill just to check the mail felt like a monumental task. (We didn't have email at the time.) I knew I had everything I needed, yet I felt down and out at times. I also felt isolated from the "real world," a "successful" career and socialization.

I was often bombarded by the pressures of daily chores, the upkeep, and trying to keep Dad busy, feeling productive and giving him things to do that gave his life purpose. It worked. Dad felt so fulfilled, he often claimed the accident was the best thing that could have happened to him. The injury introduced him to the realm of meditation from eastern philosophy, something he would have never considered if he had remained "normal."

By embracing the isolation and solitude, he transformed his life and found answers to his deepest questions in the silence devoid of hoopla from the external noice of the outside world.

My dad lived with us until he reached the age of 88 when we needed to sadly admit him into a hospital in 2020. By that time he was showing signs of dementia. He and I hardly spent a day away from each other's company since his 1984 injury. It was a struggle to be separated from him for the first time in decades that last year when he was unable to communicate his needs, no longer being cared for at home but rather at a nursing home during the onset of COVID when I was not allowed to visit him.

A year and a half later, he passed away. Devastatingly, because he could not communicate and in addition to the dementia, my sister and I learned he was physically abused (more than twelve uninvestigated bruises on his body) at the facility and inflicted with delirium from the medications—medications he would have never agreed to because he was a huge proponent of natural remedies -- like silence and solitude found in this book. See, Dad's motto went from "don't just sit there, do something" prior to his injury in 1984 when he was a busy and active engineer to "don't just do something, sit there" after his injury while recovering.

Dad used the meditation techniques found inside this book to not only cope with multiple losses but to live happily-ever-after. It will help you transform isolation and loneliness into something you hold sacred.

> *"I don't suffer from insanity. I enjoy every moment of it." ~Dad*

If you've had a few speed bumps, hurdles, hills or even mountains to climb, remember, they are temporary and they can be worked through. Walking in nature and embracing solitude can lift you from those slumps. The more you reconnect with your natural self, the stronger you become. Silence offers a chance to recharge and rediscover your life's purpose.

It took me a while, but I finally realized that what we say to ourselves matters a great deal. The internal dialogue that runs through our minds can either lift us up or drag us down. This book is designed to help you develop the skills to find value in who you are and ensure that what you say to yourself uplifts you and connects you to your greater SELF (Sacred Energy Life Force). You can find strength in solitude.

The mindful ideas presented in this book can be practiced by anyone, at any time, and in any location. It doesn't matter who you are or what limitations, political, or religious leanings you might have. In today's divided landscape, finding ways to "stay calm and carry on" is essential. You don't have to wait until you are isolated from the rest of the crowd to begin this journey, you can embrace silence now.

> *When you visualize a special place or imagine a serene scene, it's like a dream where you are truly present. From there you can be who you truly are.*
>
> ~ Janine

This book is my way of sharing that journey with you, offering ideas on therapeutic writing exercises and suggestions to help you find peace, joy, and self-discovery in your own life.

Through embracing silence, I've learned to distinguish between my immediate reactions and my deeper consciousness. This helps me avoid unnecessary actions and focus on what truly matters. Tranquility allows me to organize my thoughts and align with my authentic self. It helps me stay connected with nature and with the collective plan, finding harmony and releasing worries.

Silence helps you write purposefully, understand your dreams, and recognize the dual identities within you—the ego trying to survive and the soul connected to universal love.

As humans, we are capable of so much. To keep peace within, remind yourself not to take on more than you can handle. You are not responsible for solving all the world's problems but can focus on what is closest to you. Sometimes, just getting out of bed, getting the mail, and smiling at someone is enough for the day. Taking each day as it comes, you will eventually see that you have accomplished a lot, simply by being present and trying your best. Use these moments of solitude to connect with your greater SELF. This inner sacred space will give you answers and help you see with clarity. Embrace the silence, and you will find the strength and wisdom within you.

This book is intended to guide you to develop a nurturing internal dialogue, serving as a gentle reminder to find value in who you are. It will show you how to ensure that what you say to yourself uplifts you and connects you to your true self. Embrace the power of isolation, and discover the beautiful strength within your sacred energy life force.

Imagine taking a break from the noise—turning off the bad news, stepping away from social media, and just being with yourself. Even if it's temporary, it's a way to collect your thoughts and explore your true self --your sacred energy life force. Silence is golden when you use it to your advantage.

Therapeutic Writing Session: Share a story about a time when you found peace and clarity during a silent retreat or a quiet walk in nature. If you haven't yet, try it!

Suggestion: Take a few minutes each day to sit in silence, listen to your breath, and enjoy the tranquility.

ABOUT JANINE VANCE

Janine Vance has dedicated her life to the exploration of metaphysics, philosophy, and the power of storytelling. Her journey is marked by a deep belief in the transformative power of shared experiences and the importance of history being written by those most impacted by it.

Vance's professional experience and publications reflect her commitment to spiritual growth and self-discovery. Her publications, from her first book *Twins Found in a Box: Adapting to Adoption* (2003) to one of her later books *Going Back to Zen* (2018), offer insights into her spiritual journey and her exploration of metaphysics.

Janine's passion for storytelling is evident in her work as an author and her passion for book development and design. She has assisted more than fifty writers in becoming published authors, helping them share their unique stories with the world. Her books, described as "uplifting," "peaceful," and "a great help when things are spiraling," serve as a testament to her belief in the power of storytelling.

Vance's spiritual career, marked by her exploration of metaphysics, philosophy, and storytelling since 1998, serves as an inspiration for those seeking to embark on their own journey of self-discovery. Janine's spiritual journey is underpinned by her academic pursuits in the field of metaphysics since 2003 when she first became a Metaphysical minister. She holds a Ministerial Doctor of Philosophy Degree specializing in Conscious-Centered Living (2019).

Janine served as her dad's primary caregiver from 1984 until his death in 2021 at the age of 90. She continues to provide ideas for therapeutic writing and solace through her writings and philosophy.

Janine appreciates your supportive comments and reviews.

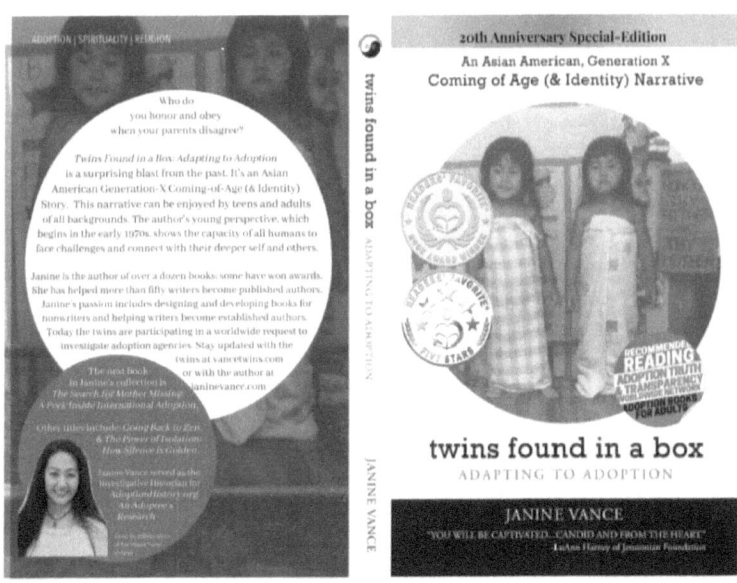

A PERSONAL CHILDHOOD STORY (2003)

Amazon Review: "I was drawn in right from the beginning, with the descriptions of all the 80's styles and awkward teenage years. It reads like a fiction book with so many interesting details. The descriptions of the family dynamic are given from a very objective viewpoint so the reader really grasps how unfair the situation was without any hint of anger or bitterness in the words. Aside from the adoption community, I really think the spiritual community would be enriched by reading this story. Most of all, I absolutely LOVE the end, when the author talks about her spiritual growth, expanding to other spiritual ideas, and especially how she came to see the deeper meaning in all of those experiences. The last few chapters are so incredibly powerful! By the end, I felt like my spirit was bursting with joy that she came to such a beautiful place of healing and that she generously shared that with others. I Loved it!!!" For fun, visit www.vancetwins.com.

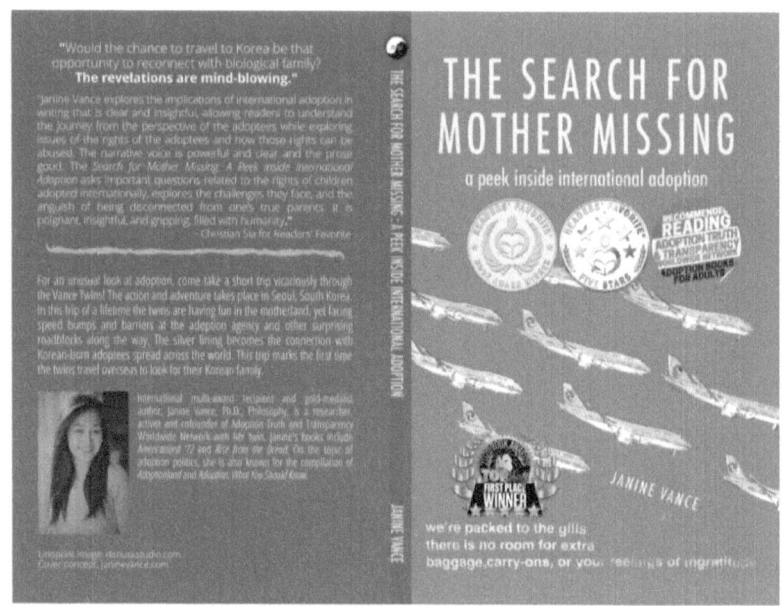

COME WITH US! LET'S GO TO SEOUL, SOUTH KOREA!"

"Did you miss the anniversary gathering commemorating 50 years of overseas adoption in South Korea? In this contemporary tale detailing a two-week trip that explores intercountry adoption from South Korea, the Vance Twins travel to their birth city of Seoul in search of their Korean family. Awarded First Place in the genre of Adventure by Top Shelf Books. Awarded Gold and five stars in the Non-Fiction Adventure Category by Readers' Favorite International Book Contest.

Amazon Review: *"I read the ENTIRE book from front to back in 2 days! That is RECORD time for me! As a Korean Adoptee, and an aspiring author, it is important to me to learn about other adoptees' stories, international adoption and our "motherland". I learned more about Korea and International adoption from this book than I've ever learned in 36 years of life. The information was really enlightening. So much of what I was told or assumed as a child about Korea was not true. So much of what I suspected as I've gotten older was true."*

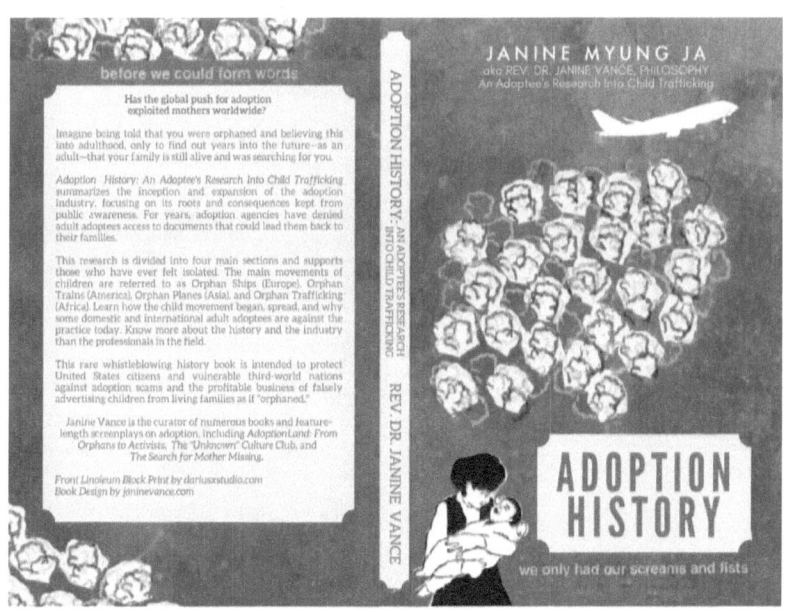

ADOPTIONHISTORY.ORG: OF, BY & FOR THE PEOPLE

You need to know what adoption agencies refuse to tell you about the growing and exploding child migration movement that has ignored the rights of families all over the world. This unconventional history book has been called mind-blowing by fellow human-rights activists. The main movements of children are organized into four sections and referred to as orphan ships (Europe), orphan trains (America), orphan planes (Asia), and orphan trafficking (Africa). Fellow adoptee rights activists have called the book "Revealing," "Enlightening," and "Mindblowing." Also available on audiobook. This version was awarded five stars and won silver at the Readers' Favorite International Book Award Ceremony in the Non-Fiction Gov/Politics Category. If you're adopted, be sure to take the "Only in Adoption" survey for domestic, late-discovery, transracial, and overseas adoptees at www.AdoptionHistory.org.

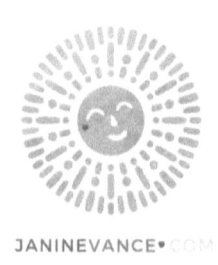

JANINEVANCE.COM

FOR WRITING SABBATICALS,
FIND JANINE AT
PERSONAL & PHILOSOPHY:
WWW.JANINEVANCE.COM

FUN WITH VANCE TWINS:
WWW.VANCETWINS.COM

POLITICS & HISTORY:
WWW.ADOPTIONHISTORY.ORG